MANIFESTATIONS OF CYTOMEGALOVIRUS INFECTION

Edited by **Patricia Price, Nandini Makwana** and **Samantha Brunt**

Manifestations of Cytomegalovirus Infection
http://dx.doi.org/10.5772/50832
Edited by Patricia Price, Nandini Makwana and Samantha Brunt

Contributors

Matthew Bates, Alimuddin Zumla, Ana Corona Nakamura, Martha Arias Merino, John Tomtishen, Patricia Price, Ilka Boin, Shin-Ichi Usami, Prakash Vishnu, David M. Aboulafia

Published by InTech
Janeza Trdine 9, 51000 Rijeka, Croatia

Publishing Process Manager Oliver Kurelic
Typesetting InTech DTP Team
Cover InTech Design Team

Additional hard copies can be obtained from orders@intechopen.com

Manifestations of Cytomegalovirus Infection, Edited by Patricia Price, Nandini Makwana and Samantha Brunt
p. cm.
ISBN 978-953-51-1116-0

For EU product safety concerns:
IN TECH d.o.o., Prolaz Marije Krucifikse Kozulić 3, 51000 Rijeka, Croatia,
info@intechopen.com or visit our website at intechopen.com.

Meet the editors

Patricia Price, Editor
The focus of my work is HIV disease - specifically the consequences of beginning ART with low CD4 T-cell counts. This has included studies of Immune Restoration Diseases associated with opportunistic infections that are common in the developing world. We showed that poor control of HCV replication marks Indonesian patients experiencing relapses of HCV disease on ART. A larger study in Jakarta will correlate "the footprint" of chronic CMV infection with clinical endpoints in patients beginning ART. We are also studying CMV immunology at Royal Perth Hospital/University of Western Australia. We are addressing the role of CMV in immunological aging – comparing the footprint of CMV in HIV patients and renal transplant recipients with that seen in healthy individuals of a similar age.

Nandini Makwana, Editor
I am pursuing a PhD at the University of Western Australia, and my interest is in the effects of Cytomegalovirus on Natural Killer cells and adaptive immune response in renal transplant patients. I have expertise in tissue culture work, and have worked on Japanese Encephalitits, West Nile and Bagaza virus in National Institute of Virology, India, which is also a WHO collaborating centre for Arboviruses and Haemorrhagic fever reference and research. I have also done in-vitro screening of anti-HIV compounds and microbicides at the National AIDS Research Institute, India, and have gained expertise on setting up human cervical explant cultures. My area of interest is virology and immunology but I also hold a postgraduate certificate degree in clinical research and clinical data management.

Samantha Brunt, Editor
Following on from my B.Sc in biomedical science which was completed during 2012, my PhD work focuses on Cytomegalovirus antibody production in HIV patients. This is an interest of a larger project investigating CMV immunity and how it relates to accelerated aging and increased prevalence of age associated diseases, such as cardiovascular disease. I am continuing investigations into the 'footprint' CMV infection leaves on a person's immune system, focusing on B-cell activation and also prevalence of auto-antibodies relative to CMV antibody. My honours work demonstrated a correlation of high CMV antibody titres and increased risk of cardiovascular disease in HIV patients stable on therapy.

Contents

Preface

CMV is a prevalent viral pathogen that rarely causes recognisable symptoms in immunocompetent hosts. CMV is the strangest virus. It has 200 genes but needs only 30 to replicate. It infects everyone but few people have heard of it. We carry it all our lives but it can rarely be isolated from blood. Up to 23% of CD8 T-cells can be specific for CMV in older healthy adults, despite undetectable viral load. CMV-specific T-cells have a "worn out" phenotype, likely gained from lifelong surveillance of persistent CMV which re-awakens in response to stresses or inflammation.

CMV causes distinct patterns of disease in different classes of immunodeficient patients. This includes retinitis in HIV patients, pneumonitis after transplantation and deafness in babies. This book includes chapters focussing on different groups of individuals at risk.

CMV reactivation (in previously seropositive recipients) or primary infection (in any recipient) is the most common infectious complication in renal transplantation. In the 1970's one in three recipients experienced pathologies associated with CMV. In most countries, prophylaxis (valganciclovir) is routinely administered for 12-26 weeks after transplantation. However CMV remains a significant cause of graft loss and the optimal duration of prophylaxis is unclear. In the longer term, CMV reactivations are implicated in deterioration in renal function, cardiovascular disease and perhaps type II diabetes.

CMV has also been anecdotally linked with cardiovascular disease and in vitro studies show increased expression of adhesion molecules in endothelial tissues infected with CMV. One study linked T-cell responses to CMV with cardiovascular symptoms (atherosclerosis) in HIV patients. CMV-DNA has been found in tissues removed during surgery for abdominal aortic aneurysm and CMV seropositivity is more frequent in coronary artery disease requiring surgery. In HIV patients, stronger T-cell responses to CMV (considered an indication of exposure to CMV rather protection) associate with cardiovascular changes.

In this book we also consider CMV in the developing world where it has been comprehensively ignored. However this must change as ART is rolled out for HIV patients worldwide and transplantation becomes feasible in South America, Africa and Asia. We need to understand the dynamic role of CMV in these populations.

Finally we need to understand how infection of so few cells with CMV has such dramatic effects. Perhaps CMV has effects even broader than we realise. CMV is a highly evolved virus. The last chapter discusses the need for novel therapeutics to reduce the impact of CMV infection in at risk groups.

Patricia Price
University of Western Australia, Australia

Nandini Makwana
Pune University, India

Samantha Brunt
University of Western Australia, Australia

Chapter 1

Hearing Loss in Children with Congenital Cytomegalovirus Infection

Satoshi Iwasaki and Shin-ich Usami

Additional information is available at the end of the chapter

http://dx.doi.org/10.5772/56160

1. Introduction

Sensorineural hearing loss (SNHL) is a common birth defect. The genetic origins of SNHL can be identified in half of the prelingual cases; in the others, SNHL is caused by environmental or unidentified genetic factors. The most common environmental cause of SNHL is congenital cytomegalovirus (CMV) infection. CMV is also the most common cause of intrauterine and congenital viral infection, affecting 0.5% to 2.5% of all live neonates [1]. While 90% of CMV-infected children are asymptomatic at birth, 10% of those exhibit clinically apparent sequelae at birth, including SNHL, mental retardation, motor disability, and microcephaly [1-4]. Recent studies have revealed that children with asymptomatic congenital CMV infection are at risk of late-onset SNHL and/or deterioration of SNHL during early childhood. These developments may not appear until months or even years following birth. The frequency of SNHL associated with asymptomatic congenital CMV infection reportedly ranges from 13% to 24% [5-9]. Although asymptomatic CMV infection is associated with a lower incidence of SNHL than symptomatic CMV infection, SNHL caused by congenital CMV often remains undiagnosed because maternal screening for CMV infection is not routinely conducted and the detection of SNHL during newborn hearing screening (NHS) tests is difficult [7, 10].

Hearing loss is detected in approximately 50% of children with symptomatic congenital CMV infection. In 66% of these patients, hearing loss will deteriorate [3, 11]. Children with symptomatic congenital CMV infection are easily identified at birth. In children with symptomatic infection, intrauterine growth retardation and petechiae have been associated with the development of hearing loss [12]. SNHL is diagnosed in 7%–25% of children with asymptomatic congenital CMV infection. Rates of delayed-onset SNHL, progressive SNHL, and improvement of SNHL are reported to be 11%–18%, 23%–62%, and 23% – 47%, respectively [5-9].

Thus, the incidence of asymptomatic CMV infection and resulting SNHL may be higher, making it the leading cause of SNHL in children. Treatment of children with congenital CMV infection can prevent late-onset SNHL and/or deterioration of SNHL during early childhood. Cochlear implantation is also effective for the development of speech perception and auditory skills for deaf children with congenital CMV infection. Therefore, early identification of congenital CMV infection is very important.

2. Epidemiology of hearing-impaired children with congenital CMV infection

Of the 12,599 pregnant women included in a prospective study [13] conducted where from June 1996 to December 2003, maternal ages were as follows: <20 years, 1.6%; 20–24 years, 14.7%; 25–29 years, 41.4%; 30–34 years, 28.6%; 35–39 years, 7.9%; and >40 years, 0.8%. The annual seropositivity rate decreased over the 8-year study period, particularly during the last 4 years. The seropositivity rate of CMV immunoglobulin G (IgG) antibody was 75.3% in the sample as a whole. The seronegativity rate was 23.6%, and the percentage of cases borderline positive for IgG antibody was 1%. The seronegativity rate of CMV IgM antibody was 94.8% in the sample as a whole. The seropositivity rate was 2.2%, and 3% of cases were borderline positive for CMV IgM antibody. During the study period, in the cases positive for IgM antibody (n = 146), borderline positive for IgM antibody (n = 73), and borderline positive for IgG antibody (n = 14) and in cases with seroconversion of IgG antibody (n = 3), neonatal urine was analyzed for CMV DNA. Seroconversion of CMV IgG antibody occurred in 0.32% of the 929 cases negative for IgG antibody. Congenital CMV infection was identified in 18 infants by polymerase chain reaction (PCR) analysis of urine. Follow-up was conducted in these cases.

The symptoms at birth and sequelae observed during the first 6 months of life in the 18 children with congenital CMV infection are shown in Table 1. Among these infants, 2 children (11.1%) were symptomatic and the remaining 16 (88.9%) were asymptomatic. In this study, newborn infants were considered symptomatic if central nervous system involvement such as microcephaly or ventricular dilatation was detected. SNHL was detected in 1 child (50%) with symptomatic infection and in 4 children (25%) with asymptomatic infection. Profound unilateral SNHL had developed in the child with symptomatic infection. In the 4 children with asymptomatic infection, the severity of SNHL varied from mild unilateral loss to profound bilateral loss. Of the 4 children, unilateral SNHL was identified in 3 (75%). Mild unilateral SNHL occurred in 2 children (66.7%), and profound unilateral loss occurred in 1 child (33.3%). Profound bilateral SNHL occurred in 1 child with asymptomatic infection. The unilateral hearing loss in case 1 was detected by a neonatal automatic auditory brainstem response (ABR) screener. SNHL in the other 3 children was detected by conventional ABR. Table 2 shows a summary of the findings from longitudinal audiological evaluations in the 5 children with asymptomatic congenital CMV infection. On subsequent audiological testing, delayed-onset SNHL was detected in 2 children who had passed the newborn hearing screening (NHS) test (1 bilateral and 1 unilateral). Two cases (40%) had progressive hearing loss and 2 (40%) had

http://dx.doi.org/10.5772/56160

improvement of hearing loss from the initial abnormal ABR (profound unilateral loss and profound bilateral loss, respectively).

	Symptoms	Audiologic examinations
Case 1	Not found	Automatic ABR: unilateral REFER ABR: unilateral moderate hearing loss
Case 2	Not found	ABR: unilateral moderate hearing loss
Case 3	Not found	ABR: unilateral profound hearing loss
Case 4	Not found	ABR: bilateral severe hearing loss
Case 5	Not found	Automatic ABR: bilateral PASS
Case 6-16	Not found	ABR: normal
Case 17	Microcephaly Ventricular dilatation	ABR: unilateral profound hearing loss
Case 18	Microcephaly Ventricular dilatation Heart anomaly	ABR: normal

ABR: auditory brainstem response. This table is cited from reference [11].

Table 1. Initial symptoms and audiologic results during the first 6 months of life in 18 children with congenital CMV infection.

	Initial hearing loss	Results of follow-up audiologic examination			Outcome
		Age	Hearing loss	Characteristic	
Case 1	Unilateral moderate (Unilateral REFER)	36 mo	Bilateral profound	Delayed-onset Progressive	Cochlear implantation (39 mo)
Case 2	Unilateral moderate	53 mo	Unilateral moderate	Fluctuating	Normal speech development
Case 3	Unilateral profound	53 mo	Unilateral mild	Fluctuating Improvement	Normal speech development
Case 4	Bilateral severe	17 mo	Normal	Fluctuating Improvement	Normal speech development
Case 5	Normal (Bilateral PASS)	26 mo	Bilateral profound	Delayed-onset Progressive	Cochlear implantation (29 mo)

SNHL: sensorineural hearing loss. This table is cited from reference [11].

Table 2. Results of longitudinal audiologic examinations in 5 children with SNHL caused by asymptomatic CMV infection.

In this prospective study, the rates of delayed-onset SNHL, progressive SNHL, and improvement of SNHL were 12%, 40%, and 40%, respectively. Although a low rate of fetal CMV infection was observed, the results of the present study regarding the rate of SNHL are in accordance with the findings of those previous studies. The prevalence of congenital CMV infection is affected by the socioeconomic and geographic differences, but it seems to be no differences on characteristics of hearing loss induced by congenital CMV infection.

Because they develop later, both delayed-onset and progressive hearing loss frequently remain undiagnosed during universal newborn hearing screening (NHS) test [7, 10]. The 1994 Joint Committee on Infant Hearing [14] pointed out that additional hearing evaluations after universal NHS are required to detect delayed-onset hearing loss. Combined neonatal screening for CMV infection and repeated auditory evaluation should be considered, particularly for children with asymptomatic congenital CMV infection. Counseling of pregnant women on prevention of CMV infection is also important.

2.1. Retrospective study of congenital CMV infection

Hearing loss in children with congenital CMV infection often presents at birth; however, in many instances, it may develop after months or even years. One report stated that children with normal hearing at 6 months of age develop hearing loss at a rate of approximately 1% per year; the cumulative risk of late-onset hearing loss is substantial (6.9%) in a population of infants with asymptomatic congenital CMV infection [15]. Speech is often delayed in children with bilateral hearing loss. For cases of severe bilateral SNHL, Ogawa et al. [16] reported that congenital CMV infection could be diagnosed through the detection of CMV DNA in the dried umbilical cord. In addition, genetic defects (particularly those related to *GJB2*) were identified in 15% and 30% of the children, respectively. However, the etiology of pediatric SNHL, including mild to moderate and unilateral SNHL, remains uncertain. In a study of congenital CMV infection retrospectively diagnosed by the detection of CMV DNA extracted from dried umbilical cord specimens, the prevalence of CMV in children with unilateral or bilateral SNHL was investigated. In many of these cases, SNHL developed several months or even years after birth.

In total, 134 patients (70 males and 64 females) with bilateral (n = 46; 34.3%) or unilateral (n = 88; 65.7%) SNHL were evaluated. These cases were referred to the Department of Otolaryngology, Shinshu University School of Medicine from May 2008 to September 2009 (Table 3) [17]. The age of these children ranged from 1 month to 138 months (mean age: 37.7 ± 36.2 months). In children with bilateral SNHL, both genetic testing for deafness and CMV DNA analysis were performed. For children with unilateral SNHL, CMV DNA analysis and genetic testing for gene mutations of *GJB2, Mitochondrial1555* were performed. Objective audiometric evaluation was performed for each patient using ABR and auditory steady-state evoked response systems (MASTER 580-NAVPRO; NIHON KOHDEN Co., Ltd, Tokyo, Japan). Behavioral audiological tests and/or pure-tone audiometry were also performed. Hearing levels were classified into 2 categories on the basis of the severity of hearing loss in the worse ear as severe (>70 dB) to profound (>90 dB) and mild (20–40 dB) to moderate (41–70 dB). Follow-up hearing assessments were performed at intervals of 6–12 months. Progressive hearing loss was defined as a decrease in hearing of ≥10 dB at 1 or more frequencies. Fluctuating hearing loss was defined as a decrease in hearing of >10 dB followed by an improvement of >10 dB at 1 or more frequencies. To analyze congenital CMV infection, CMV DNA quantitative PCR (qPCR) analysis was performed. Prior to qPCR analysis, total DNA, including genomic DNA and CMV DNA, was extracted from preserved dried umbilical cords. The results of this study revealed that in 9.0% (12/134) of children, SNHL could be attributed to congenital CMV infection. CMV DNA from preserved umbilical cords was detected in 8.7% (4/46) of children with bilateral SNHL and 9.1% (8/88) of those with unilateral SNHL. Congenital CMV infection caused bilateral severe-to-profound SNHL, bilateral mild-to-moderate SNHL, unilateral severe-to-profound SNHL, and unilateral mild-to-moderate SNHL in 14.3% (4/28), 0% (0/18), 9.6% (7/73), and 6.7% (1/15) of hearing-impaired children, respectively. This study also revealed that both congenital and late-onset SNHL could be caused by congenital CMV infection.

Hearing loss	**Gender**	**Hearing level**	**Severe-profound HL**		**Mild-moderate HL**	
	(n)	**(dB)**	**n**	**Diagnostic age**	**n**	**Diagnostic age**
Total (N=134)	M: 70, F: 64		101 (75.4%)	34.4±34.7 mo	33 (24.6%)	48.8±38.7 mo
Bilateral HL (N=46)	M: 31, F: 15	71.8 dB [R] 71.7 dB [L]	28 (20.9%)	16.6±19.9 mo	18 (13.4%)	11.1±39.1 mo
Unilateral HL (N=88)	M: 39, F: 49	89.5 dB (W) 13.6 dB (B)	72 (54.5%)	41.2±36.6 mo	15 (11.2%)	40.3±36.8 mo

HL: hearing loss. Diagnostic age: age diagnosed as hearing loss.

M: male, F: female. R: right, L: left. B: better ear, W: worse ear. This table is cited from reference [16].

Table 3. Summary of characteristics of children with bilateral or unilateral hearing loss.

Table 4 shows the clinical characteristics of 12 children in whom CMV DNA was identified. Of these 12 children, bilateral SNHL was detected in 4 and unilateral SNHL in 8. All 4 children with bilateral SNHL had late-onset profound SNHL. Hearing fluctuation and PASS at the NHS test were confirmed in 3 children (75%). Of the 8 children with unilateral SNHL, detectable defects were confirmed in 2 children. Hearing fluctuation was detected in only 1 child (12.5%). No inner ear anomaly was found in any of the 8 children with unilateral SNHL.

Retrospective diagnosis of congenital CMV infection is important to improve our understanding of the etiology of pediatric SNHL. In previous reports (Table 5), the frequency of congenital CMV infection in children with bilateral SNHL has varied from 3% to 36% because of variations in parameters (number of subjects, severity of SNHL) and methods [CMV IgM testing, DNA urinalysis, DNA from dried blood spots (DBS) in Guthrie cards] [19-24]. In 2 Japanese studies based on the retrospective diagnostic method of analysis of preserved dried umbilical cords, congenital CMV infection was detected in 10%–12% of children with bilateral SNHL [25, 26];

however, these studies included few subjects (10–26 cases). In children with unilateral SNHL, CMV DNA from preserved umbilical cords was detected in 9.1% (8/88). The frequency of congenital CMV infection was similar in children with unilateral and bilateral SNHL. It has been speculated that approximately 10% of SNHL in children is caused by congenital CMV infection. Few reports have examined the frequency of congenital CMV infection using retrospective diagnostic methods in children with unilateral SNHL. However, using the CMV DNA detection method, 25% (1/4) [16] and 19% (8/42) [19] of children with unilateral SNHL were diagnosed with congenital CMV infection.

Case no.	Sex	Diagnostic age	Bilateral/ Unilateral	Severity	Average HL (R/L: dB)	Onset	NHS
1	F	60 mo	Bilateral	Profound	87.5/108.8	Late	Pass
2	F	52 mo	Bilateral	Profound	87.5/110.0	Late	Pass
3	M	50 mo	Bilateral	Profound	100.0/100.0	Late	Pass
4	M	62 mo	Bilateral	Profound	110.0/46.3	Likely late	–
5	M	6 mo	Unilateral	Profound	32.5/103.8	Congenital	Refer (L)
6	M	65 mo	Unilateral	Profound	107.5/17.5	Unknown	–
7	M	50 mo	Unilateral	Profound	6.3/100.0	Unknown	–
8	F	98 mo	Unilateral	Profound	110.0/15.0	Unknown	–
9	F	55 mo	Unilateral	Profound	15.0/92.5	Late	Pass
10	F	2 mo	Unilateral	Profound	90.0/18.3	Congenital	Refer (R)
11	M	80 mo	Unilateral	Severe	13.3/70.0	Unknown	–
12	F	44 mo	Unilateral	Moderate	15.0/58.3	Late	Pass

F: female, M: male. Mo: month. HL: hearing loss. R: right, L: left. NHS: newborn hearing screening.
Diagnostic age: age diagnosed as hearing loss. This table is cited from reference [16].

Table 4. Clinical data of CMV DNA-positive children

2.2. Genetic hearing loss and congenital CMV infection

Genetic testing for deafness has become valuable for precise diagnosis of hearing loss. The most frequently implicated gene in nonsyndromic hearing loss is *GJB2*, the most prevalent gene responsible for congenital hearing loss worldwide. *GJB2, SLC26A4, CDH23*, and mitochondrial 12s ribosomal RNA (rRNA) are the other major genes that cause hearing loss in Japan. One study stated that genetic mutations were responsible for deafness in 40%–45% of children with congenital hearing loss [27]. In our study [17], 10 gene mutations associated with deafness (*GJB2*, n = 7; *SLC26A4*, n = 3) were identified in 21.7% (10/46) of children with bilateral SNHL. In children with bilateral severe-to-profound SNHL, gene mutations causing deafness

http://dx.doi.org/10.5772/56160

Reference	Year	Subjects	CMV positive rate			Diagnostic methods	Country
			Total	Bilateral	Unilateral		
Barbi et al. [19]	2003	> 40 dBHL	9/79 (11.4%)	1/37 (2.7%)	8/42 (19%)	DBS, qPCR	Italy
Ogawa et al. [16]	2007	> 20dB, nonsyndromic SNHL	10/67 (10.5%)	9/63 (14.3%)	1/4 (25%)	US, PCR	Japan
Samileh et al. [21]	2008	> 40 dBHL	33/95 (34.7%)	NR/75	NR/20	Cerologic test	Iran
Stehel et al. [22]	2008	NHS refer	16/256 (6%)	16/256 (6%)	NR	DNA from urine	USA
Walter et al. [43]	2008	unexplained SNHL	8/35 (22.9%)	NR	NR	DSS, qPCR	UK
Mizuno et al. [44]	2008	only bilateral	3/45 (6.7%)	3/45 (6.7%)	0	UC, qPCR	Japan
Jakubikova et al. [20]	2009	> 60 dBHL, NHS refer	4/71 (5.6%)	4/55 (7.3%)	0/16 (0%)	Cerologic test	Slovak Re.
Boudewyns et al. [45]	2009	NHS refer, > 20 dB	4/55 (7.3%)	NR	NR	DBS, qPCR	Belgium
Choi et al. [18]	2009	NHS refer	13/479 (2.7%)	13/479 (2.7%)	NR	DBS, qPCR	USA
Tagawa et al. [26]	2009	> 70 dB, deaf school children	3/26 (11.5%)	3/26 (11.5%)	0 (0%)	UC, qPCR	Japan
Kimani et al. [46]	2010	NHS refer	11/109 (10.1%)	8/92 (8.8%)	3/17 (17.6%)	DBS, qPCR	USA
Adachi et al. [47]	2010	NHS refer, >35dB, bilateral	13/77 (17%)	13/77 (17%)	0	US, qPCR	Japan

NR: not reported. NHS: newborn hearing screening. DBS: dried blood spot. UC: umbilical cord. qPCR: quantitative PCR. HL: hearing level. SNHL: sensorineural hearing loss. Re.: republic. This table is cited from reference [16].

Table 5. List of previous reports on children with congenital CMV nfection.

and CMV DNA positivity were detected in 32.1% (9/28) and 14.3% (4/28) of patients, respectively [17]. The diagnostic rate has been concluded to be 46.4% (13/28). If analysis of CMV DNA from preserved dried umbilical cords could be combined with genetic testing for deafness, approximately 50% of cases of bilateral severe-to-profound hearing loss in children could be detected.

Congenital CMV infection is also often diagnosed by detecting CMV DNA in urine within the first 2 weeks of life and serological testing for CMV-specific IgM antibody from mother and child [28]. In recent years, the detection of CMV DNA by retrospective methods has been more valuable not only in diagnosing congenital CMV infection during later stages of life but also in identifying children at highest risk of late-onset and progressive SNHL. Some reports have stated that DBS stored on Guthrie cards has been used for the retrospective diagnosis of congenital CMV infections [18, 29]. Similarly, preserved umbilical cords have been recently used in Japan [25, 26, 30]. The sensitivity varies widely depending on the DNA extraction method in the DBS case. Some investigators have reported sensitivities of 71%–100% and specificities of 99%–100% [19, 29]. In this study, the qPCR method and preserved umbilical cords were used because they were useful for more accurate detection of CMV DNA.

3. Diagnosis of congenital CMV infection

3.1. Detection methods

The gold standard for diagnosis of congenital CMV infection is isolation of the virus from urine or saliva in the first 2 weeks of life. However, asymptomatic congenital CMV infection in children who develop SNHL after the first 2 weeks following birth cannot be diagnosed on the basis of viral isolation from urine or saliva. Detection of CMV DNA in infant blood or the umbilical cord using PCR assays is a more feasible method for identifying children with late-onset SNHL. The method involves analysis of blood stored as DBS on Guthrie cards. In Japanese culture, the dried umbilical cord is generally stored at home as a memento of the birth. These specimens are suitable for retrospective diagnosis of congenital CMV infection. The sensitivity varied widely depending on the DNA extraction method from DBS on Guthrie cards. Some investigators reported sensitivities of 71-100% and specificities of 99-100% [19, 29]. The qPCR method and dried umbilical cord could be useful for more precise detection of CMV DNA.

3.2. Serological method

Diagnosis of symptomatic CMV infection is easier in children who display cognitive or neuromuscular abnormalities than in asymptomatic children with CMV infection. Without neonatal viral screening, the prevalence of SNHL caused by asymptomatic CMV infection remains undetermined. To diagnose primary CMV infection, a serological method has been used [31]. Pregnant women who test positive for CMV IgG seroconversion or CMV IgM antibody may transmit the virus to the fetus. Production of IgM antibody persists for 6–9 months [28]; therefore, a CMV IgM-positive result alone does not accurately predict the risk of fetal infection.

3.3. Detection of CMV DNA from umbilical cord

For the detection of congenital CMV infection, CMV DNA qPCR analysis was performed. Prior to qPCR analysis, total DNA, including genomic DNA and CMV DNA, was extracted from preserved dried umbilical cords. The procedure is as follows. Each 5-mm tissue section was incubated in a lysis buffer containing proteinase K and incubated overnight at 56°C. Total DNA was extracted using the DNeasy® Blood & Tissue Kit (Qiagen GmbH, Hilden, Germany), according to the manufacturer's instructions. The total amount of DNA was measured using the Qubit® Fluorometer with Quant-iT™ dsDNA BR Assay Kit (Life technologies-Invitrogen, Carlsbad, CA, USA). Total DNA (10 pg) was analyzed using the Step One Real-Time PCR System (Applied Biosystems, Foster City, CA, USA) and TaqMan® Universal Master Mix II (Applied Biosystems). The qPCR primers and TaqMan® probe used for CMV DNA qPCR analysis were as follows: US14-1F: 5′-ACGTCCACGTTAGGATGAGG-3′, US14-1R: 5′-GTATGTGGCGCTTCTCTCGT-3′, and US14-1 TaqMan probe: 5′-FAM- AACCTGTGCACCACAGCGCC -TAMRA-3′. To quantify the input DNA amount in each sample, qPCR of each genomic region was also performed using the following primers and TaqMan® probe: GJB2-2F: 5′-ACGTCCACGT-TAGGATGAGG-3′, GJB2-2: 5′-GTATGTGGCGCTTCTCTCGT-3′, and GJB2-2 TaqMan probe: 5′-FAM- AACCTGTGCACCACAGCGCC -TAMRA-3′. The initial preheating steps were performed for 2 min at 50°C and 10 min at 95°C. Following this, qPCR was performed for 43 cycles of 15 s at 95°C and 60 s at 60°C. After qPCR analysis, relative CMV concentrations in each sample were evaluated as ΔCt (delta cycle threshold), which was calculated by determining the threshold cycle of CMV qPCR minus that of *GJB2* qPCR. The invader assay described by Abe [32] was used for genetic testing for deafness.

4. Treatment for hearing loss induced by congenital CMV infection

4.1. Cochlear implantation in children deafened by symptomatic CMV infection

Cochlear implantation for the correction of congenital deafness is an effective way to ensure the development of speech recognition. Cochlear implantation in children deafened by symptomatic CMV infection has been reported [33, 34]. The prognosis of children with symptomatic CMV infection is worse than that of those with asymptomatic CMV infection with regard to cognitive and neurological development. It has been suggested that cochlear implantation should be contraindicated for infants with symptomatic CMV infection and deafness because they are less likely to develop spoken language [35]. In contrast, other reports [33, 34] have suggested that cochlear implantation may improve quality of life, even if progress is slower or lesser than that expected in congenitally deaf children not infected with CMV. Pyman et al. [35] suggested that the prognosis in terms of linguistic outcome after cochlear implantation is poorer for CMV-infected deaf children than for other congenitally deaf children because of coexisting central disorders. Wide variation in speech perception and intelligibility after cochlear implantation has also been reported in children deafened by symptomatic CMV infection [33]. In that report, poor development in these areas was observed in 50% of children with symptomatic CMV infection, whereas development similar to that in congenitally deaf children not infected with CMV was evident in 31% of children and development better than that in noninfected congenitally deaf children was evident in 19% of children. In addition, a recent study has shown that deafness caused by symptomatic congenital CMV infection associated with motor and cognitive delays is not a contraindication for cochlear implantation. Early diagnosis of hearing loss and subsequent cochlear implantation is important for successful speech perception [34].

4.2. Cochlear implantation in children deafened by asymptomatic CMV infection

The effectiveness of cochlear implantation in children deafened as a result of symptomatic congenital CMV infection has been evaluated by various groups, but there are only limited outcome data for deaf children with asymptomatic CMV infection. Children with asymptomatic congenital CMV infection have a better prognosis than symptomatic children, but it is difficult to evaluate the SNHL because children with asymptomatic congenital CMV infection are at risk of development of delayed onset SNHL and progressive SNHL. As a result, they are also at risk of late-onset learning difficulties and/or progressive learning difficulties.

A prospective study was conducted on deaf children with asymptomatic CMV infection to assess the development of speech perception and auditory skills. This study examined 2 deaf infants before and after cochlear implantation using the Infant/Toddler Meaningful Auditory Integration Scale (IT-MAIS) [36]. Vocalization behavior in case 1 was observed 6 months after implementation and showed slow improvement but finally overtook after 36 months. After 3 months of cochlear implant use, the 2 children responded to speech and environmental sounds in everyday situations and interpreted sounds in a meaningful way. They continued to improve at 36 months postoperatively. IT-MAIS scores in these 2 children were similar to the mean scores in the 5 congenitally deaf children without CMV infection. No difference was observed in the effect of early cochlear implantation for deafness induced by CMV infection between the groups of children. Another group reported that significant improvement in auditory and language skills could be achieved in cochlear implanted children with asymptomatic CMV infection, but they did not achieve the same levels of outcome as congenitally deaf children without CMV infection [37]. They found a wide variation in the outcome of cochlear implantation in these children and speculated that the variation is related to the degree of cognitive impairment. There are only a few studies available on outcomes of cochlear implanted children with asymptomatic CMV infection. Therefore, more studies will be needed to evaluate the effectiveness of cochlear implantation in these children.

4.3. Treatment for hearing-impaired children with congenital CMV infection

To prevent late-onset and/or deterioration of SNHL, treatment with intravenous ganciclovir (GCV) and/or oral valganciclovir (VGCV) has been recommended in children with symptomatic congenital CMV disease involving the central nervous system [38-41]. In previous reports, treatment with intravenous GCV was initiated within the first 10–14 days of life for 2–6 weeks, and GCV doses ranged from 5 to 12 mg/kg twice daily. One report revealed that in 5 of 9 children with congenital CMV infection and SNHL, treatment with intravenous GCV induced improvement of SNHL in 2 children and prevented deterioration of SNHL in 5 children [38]. Another report revealed that in 4 of 6 children with congenital CMV infection and SNHL, treatment with intravenous GCV induced improvement of SNHL in 2 children and no deterioration of SNHL in 4 children during the 21-month observation period [39]. Improvement of SNHL or maintenance of normal hearing was reported in 84% of children treated with intravenous GCV and 59% of untreated children. Deterioration of SNHL was reported in 21% of treated children and 68% of untreated children [40]. According to these reports, good results have been observed in the group of children treated with GCV. Treatment with intravenous GCV and oral VGCV can prevent the development of SNHL during an 18-month administration period [41]. Treatment with intravenous GCV has been investigated in hearing-impaired children with asymptomatic congenital CMV infection. No SNHL was found for 4 – 11 years in 12 children with asymptomatic congenital CMV infection treated with intravenous GCV, but SNHL developed in 2 of 11 untreated children [42]. Unfortunately there is no evidence for the efficacy of longer treatment with oral VGCV.

5. Conclusion

Congenital CMV infection is a major cause of bilateral and unilateral SNHL in children. In total, 9.0% of SNHL cases of unknown causes (bilateral SNHL: 8.7%, unilateral SNHL: 9.1%) are attributed to congenital CMV infection. Screening tests such as the detection of CMV DNA from preserved dried umbilical cords and genetic testing are important for the detection of SNHL in children. Using this combined methodology, detection of the cause of SNHL is possible in approximately 50% of children with hearing loss.

Cochlear implantation is effective to ensure the development of speech perception and auditory skills in deaf children with asymptomatic congenital CMV infection. No significant difference in growth of meaningful auditory integration was observed between the overall pediatric cochlear implant population not infected with CMV and that with asymptomatic CMV infection. Implementation of CMV screening models is important to prevent late-onset SNHL and deterioration of hearing loss.

Acknowledgements

These works were supported by grants for Research on Sensory and Communicative Disorders from Ministry of Health, Labour and Welfare and grants for Scientific Research (C) from Ministry of Education, Culture, Sports, Science and Technology, Tokyo, Japan.

Author details

Satoshi Iwasaki[1] and Shin-ich Usami[2*]

*Address all correspondence to: usami@shinshu-u.ac.jp

1 Department of Hearing Implant Sciences, Shinshu University School of Medicine, Matsumoto City, Japan

2 Department of Otorhinolaryngology, Shinshu University School of Medicine, Matsumoto City, Japan

References

[1] Hagay, Z. J, Biran, G, Ornoy, A, & Reece, E. A. Congenital cytomegalovirus infection: a long-standing problem still seeking a solution. Am J Obstet Gynecol (1996). , 174, 241-5.

[2] Stagno, S, Pass, R. F, Cloud, G, Britt, W. J, Henderson, R. E, Walton, P. D, et al. Primary cytomegalovirus infection in pregnancy. Incidence, transmission to fetus, and clinical outcome. JAMA (1986). , 256, 1904-8.

[3] Pass, R. F, Stagno, S, Myers, G. J, & Alford, C. A. Outcome of symptomatic congenital cytomegalovirus infection: results of long-term longitudinal follow-up. Pediatrics (1980). , 66, 758-62.

[4] Kimberlin, D. W, Lin, C. Y, Sanchez, P. J, Demmler, G. J, Dankner, W, Shelton, M, et al. Effect of ganciclovir therapy on hearing in symptomatic congenital cytomegalovirus disease involving the central nervous system: a randomized, controlled trial. J Pediatr (2003). , 143, 16-25.

[5] Yow, M. D, Williamson, D. W, Leeds, L. J, Thompson, P, Woodward, R. M, Walmus, B. F, et al. Epidemiologic characteristics of cytomegalovirus infection in mothers and their infants. Am J Obstet Gynecol (1988). , 158, 1189-95.

[6] Williamson, W. D, Demmler, G. J, Percy, A. K, & Catlin, F. I. Progressive hearing loss in infants with asymptomatic congenital cytomegalovirus infection. Pediatrics (1992). , 90, 862-6.

[7] Hicks, T, Fowler, K, Richardson, M, Dahle, A, Adams, L, & Pass, R. Congenital cytomegalovirus infection and neonatal auditory screening. J Pediatr (1993). , 123, 779-82.

[8] Fowler, K. B, Mccollister, F. P, Dahle, A. J, Boppana, S, Britt, W. J, & Pass, R. F. Progressive and fluctuating sensorineural hearing loss in children with asymptomatic congenital cytomegalovirus infection. J Pediatr (1997). , 130, 624-30.

[9] Dahle, A. J, Fowler, K. B, Wright, J. D, Boppana, S. B, Britt, W. J, & Pass, R. F. Longitudinal investigation of hearing disorders in children with congenital cytomegalovirus. J Am Acad Audiol (2000). , 11, 283-90.

[10] Fowler, K. B, Dahle, A. J, Boppana, S. B, & Pass, R. F. Newborn hearing screening: will children with hearing loss caused by congenital cytomegalovirus infection be missed? J Pediatr (1999). , 135, 60-4.

[11] Williamson, W. D, & Desmond, M. M. LaFevers N, Taber LH, Catlin FI, Weaver TG. Symptomatic congenital cytomegalovirus. Disorders of language, learning, and hearing. Am J Dis Child (1982). , 136, 902-5.

[12] Rivera, L. B, Boppana, S. B, Fowler, K. B, Britt, W. J, Stagno, S, & Pass, R. F. Predictors of hearing loss in children with symptomatic congenital cytomegalovirus infection. Pediatrics (2002). , 110, 762-7.

[13] Iwasaki, S, Yamashita, M, Maeda, M, Misawa, K, & Mineta, H. Audiological outcome of infants with congenital cytomegalovirus infection in a prospective study. Audiol Neurotol (2007). , 12, 31-6.

[14] Joint Committee on Infant Hearingposition statement. Pediatrics (1995). , 95, 152-6.

[15] Rosenthal, L. S, Fowler, K. B, Boppana, S. B, Britt, W. J, Pass, R. F, Schmid, D. S, et al. Cytomegalovirus shedding and delayed sensorineural hearing loss: results from longitudinal follow-up of children with congenital infection. Pediatr Infect Dis J (2009). , 28, 515-20.

[16] Ogawa, H, Suzutani, T, Baba, Y, Koyano, S, Nozawa, N, Ishibashi, K, et al. Etiology of severe sensorineural hearing loss in children: independent impact of congenital cytomegalovirus infection and GJB2 mutations. J Infect Dis (2007). , 195, 782-8.

[17] Furutate, S, Iwasaki, S, Nishio, S, Moteki, H, & Usami, S. Clinical profile of hearing loss in children with congenital cytpmegalovirus (CMV) infection: CMV DNA diagnosis using preserved umbilical cord. Acta Ololaryngol (2011). , 131, 976-82.

[18] Choi, K. Y, Schimmenti, L. A, Jurek, A. M, Sharon, B, Daly, K, Khan, C, et al. Detection of cytomegalovirus DNA in dried blood pots of Minnesota infants who do not pass newborn hearing screening. Pediatr Infect Dis (2009). , 28, 1095-8.

[19] Barbi M Binda SCaroppo S, Ambrosetti U, Corbetta C, Sergi P. A wider role for congenital cytomegalovirus infection in sensorineural hearing loss. Pediatr Infect Dis J (2003). , 22, 39-42.

[20] Jakubikova, J, Kabatova, Z, Pavlovcinova, G, & Profant, M. Newborn hearing screening and strategy for early detection of hearing loss in infants. Int J Pediatr Otorhinolaryngol (2009). , 73, 609-12.

[21] Samileh, N, Ahmad, S, Mohammad, F, Framarz, M, Azardokht, T, & Jomeht, E. Role of cytomegalovirus in sensorineural hearing loss of children: a case-control study Tehran, Iran. Int J Pediatr Otorhinolaryngol (2008). , 72, 203-8.

[22] Stehel, EK, Shoup, AG, & Owen, . . Newborn hearing screening and detection of congenital cytomegalovirus infection. Pediatrics 2008;121:970-5.

[23] Grosse, S. D, Ross, D. S, & Dollard, S. C. Congenital cytomegalovirus (CMV) infection as a cause of permanent bilateral hearing loss: a quantitative assessment. J Clin Virol (2008). , 41, 57-62.

[24] Foulon, I, Naessens, A, Foulon, W, Casteels, A, & Gordts, F. Hearing loss in children with congenital cytomegalovirus infection in relation to the maternal trimester in which the maternal primary infection occurred. Pediatrics (2008). e, 1123-7.

[25] Ogawa, H, Baba, Y, Suzutani, T, Inoue, N, Fukushima, E, & Omori, K. Congenital cytomegalovirus infection diagnosed by polymerase chain reaction with the use of oreserved umbilical cord in sensorineural hearing loss children. Laryngoscope (2006). , 116, 1991-4.

[26] Tagawa, M, Tanaka, H, Moriuchi, M, & Moriuchi, H. Retrospective diagnosis of congenital cytomegalovirus infection at a school for the deaf by using preserved dried umbilical cord. J Pediatr (2009). , 155, 749-51.

[27] Usami, S, Wagatsuma, M, Fukuoka, H, Suzuki, H, Tsukada, K, Nishio, S, et al. The responsible genes in Japanese deafness patients and clinical application using Invader assay. Acta Otolaryingol (2008). , 128, 446-54.

[28] Genser, B, Truschnig-wilders, M, Stunzner, D, Landini, M. D, & Halwachs-baumann, G. Evaluation of five commercial enzyme immunoassays for the detection of human cytomegalovirus-specific IgM antibodies in the absence of a commercially available gold standard. Clin Chem Lab Med (2001). , 39, 62-70.

[29] De Vries, J. C, Claas, E. C, Kroes, A. C, & Vossen, A. C. Evaluation of DNA extraction methods for dried blood spots in the diagnosis of congenital cytomegalovirus infection. J Clin Virol (2009). S, 37-42.

[30] Koyano, S, Inoue, N, Nagamori, T, Yan, H, Asanuma, H, Yagyu, K, et al. Dried umbilical cords in the retrospective diagnosis of congenital cytomegalovirus infection as a cause of developmental delays. Clin Infect Dis (2009). e, 93-5.

[31] Lazzarotto, T, Gabrielli, L, Lanari, M, Guerra, B, Bellucci, T, Sassi, M, & Landini, M. P. Congenital cytomegalovirus infection: recent advances in the diagnosis of maternal infection. Hum Immunol (2004). , 65, 410-5.

[32] Abe, S, Yamaguchi, T, & Usami, S. Application of deafness diagnostic screening panel based on deafness mutation/gene database using invader assay. Genet Test (2007). , 11, 333-40.

[33] Ramirez Inscoe JMNikolopoulos TP. Cochlear implantation in children deafened by cytomegalovirus: speech perception and speech intelligibility outcomes. Otol Neurotol (2004). , 25, 479-82.

[34] Lee, D. J, Lustig, L, Sampson, M, Chinnici, J, & Niparko, J. K. Effects of cytomegalovirus (CMV) related deafness on pediatric cochlear implant outcomes. Otolaryngol Head Neck Surg (2005). , 133, 900-5.

[35] Pyman, B, & Blamey, P. Lacy P Clark G, Dowell R. The development of speech perception in children using cochlear implants: effects of etiologic factors and delayed milestones. Am J Otol (2000). , 21, 57-61.

[36] Iwasaki, S, Nakanishi, H, Misawa, K, Tanigawa, T, & Mizuta, K. Cochlear implant in children with asymptomatic congenital cytomegalovirus infection. Audiol Neurotol (2009). , 14, 146-52.

[37] Malik, V, Bruce, I. A, Broomfield, S. J, Henderson, L, Green, K, & Ramsden, R. T. Outcome of cochlear implantation in asymptomatic congenital cytomegalovirus deafened children. Laryngoscope (2011). , 121, 1780-4.

[38] Michaels, M. G, Greenberg, D. P, Sabo, D. L, & Wald, E. R. Treatment of children with congenital cytomegalovirus infection with gancicolovir. Pediatr Infect Dis J (2003). , 22, 504-9.

[39] Kimberlin, D. W, Lin, C. Y, Sanchez, P. J, Demmler, G. J, Dankner, W, Shelton, M, et al. Effect of ganciclovir therapy on hearing in symptomatic congenital cytomegalovirus disease involving the cebtral nervous system: a randomized, controlled trial. J Pediatr (2003). , 143, 4-6.

[40] Kitajima, N, Sugaya, N, Futatani, T, Kanegane, H, Suzuki, C, Oshiro, M, et al. Ganciclovir therapy for congenital cytomegalovirus infection in six infants. Pediatr Infect Dis J (2005). , 24, 782-5.

[41] Meine Jansen CFToet MC, Rademaker CM, Ververs TH, Gerards LJ, van Loon AM. Treatment of symptomatic congenital cytomegalovirus infection with valganciclovir. J Perinat Med (2005). , 33, 363-6.

[42] Lackner, A, Acham, A, Alborno, T, Moser, M, Engele, H, Raggam, R. B, et al. Effect on hearing of ganciclovir therapy for asymptomatic congenital cytomegalovirus infection: four to 10 year follow up. J Laryngol Otol (2009). , 123, 392-6.

[43] Walter, S, Atkinson, C, Sharland, M, Rice, P, Raglan, E, Emery, V. C, et al. Congenital cytomegalovirus: association between dried blood spot viral load and hearing loss. Arch Dis Child Fetal Neonatal Ed (2008). , 93, 280-5.

[44] Mizuno, T, Sugiura, S, Kimura, H, Ando, Y, Sone, M, Nishiyama, Y, et al. Detection of cytomegalovirus DNA in preserved umbilical cords from patients with sensorineural hearing loss. Eur Arch Otorhinolaryngol (2009). , 266, 351-5.

[45] Boudewyns, A, Declau, F, Smets, K, Ursi, D, & Eyskens, F. Van den Ende J, et al. Cytomegalovirus DNA detection in Guthrie cards: role in the giagnostic work-up of childhood hearing loss. Otol Neurotol (2009). , 30, 943-9.

[46] Kimani, J. W, Buchman, C. A, Booker, J. K, Huang, B. Y, Castillo, M, Powell, C. M, et al. Seonsorineural hearing loss in a pediatric population: association of cobgenital cytomegalovirus infection with intracranial abnormalities. Arch Otolaryngol Head Neck Surg (2010). , 136, 999-1004.

[47] Adachi, N, Ito, K, Sakata, H, & Yamasoba, T. Etiology and one-year follow-up results of hearing loss identified by screening of newborn hearing in Japan. Otolaryngol Head Neck Surg (2010). , 143, 97-100.

Chapter 2

Human Cytomegalovirus (HCMV) Infection in Sub-Saharan Africa

Matthew Bates, Kunda Musonda and Alimuddin Zumla

Additional information is available at the end of the chapter

http://dx.doi.org/10.5772/54907

1. Introduction

1.1. HCMV epidemiology in Sub-Saharan Africa

1.1.1. HCMV seroprevalence

There have been over 25 published studies which present HCMV IgG seroprevalence data for sub-Saharan Africa patient groups and cohorts of healthy blood donors (Table 1). Up to eight different serology assays were used and older pre-ELISA methods might have slightly underestimated prevalence [1]. Antibodies to HCMV are generally present in high titres in seropositive individuals, so the use of different assays is unlikely to have had a major effect [2]. Hence, comparing these studies is primarily confounded by the diverse range of patient groups tested. Few studies stratify by age, or they do so using different groupings. Most of the studies use convenience samples, which do not provide accurate population-based estimates of prevalence.

The most striking observation is that HCMV primary infection appears to be endemic in young infants. A population-based study in Zambia of 460 healthy infants showed 83% HCMV seroprevalence by 18 months of age [3](Table 1). This backs up much older studies from the Gambia [4] and Nigeria [5]. This differs from the results of larger studies in the USA (n = 30,000) where HCMV seroprevalence ranges from 36% in 6–11 year-olds to 91% in those over 80 years old. The cumulative incidence of HCMV primary infection was ~1% per year from adolescence [6]. In the USA, non-white ethnicity and lower socioeconomic status (SES) were linked with 10-30 percentage point increases in seroprevalence [7]. A study of over 20,000 women in the U.K attending antenatal clinics found similar results, with increasing parity also being linked with increased HCMV seroprevalence. This supports the notion that seronegative adult women contract primary HCMV infection from children who are shedding virus [8]. Figure 1 presents a model for cumulative HCMV seroprevalence by age with respect to SES, showing more rapid uptake in low SES communities, and delayed uptake in high SES communities. Conversely an Israeli study found the effect of ethnicity persisted even when corrected for gender, education and SES [9], and high HCMV seroprevalence has been described in populations with high SES groups [10, 11].

Whilst lower SES may be the main driver for endemic infant HCMV primary infection in sub-Saharan Africa, this is not the whole story. What factors, attributable to low SES, facilitate earlier HCMV transmission? HCMV is primarily transmitted through body fluids, being shed in urine, saliva [12, 13] and breast milk [14, 15]. In Nigeria, over-crowding was significantly associated with being HCMV seropositive, but source of drinking water, place of abode and type of toilet facility were not [16]. Some individuals remain seronegative into old age - even in sub-Saharan Africa where most people are infected in infancy. Human genetic variations may block or impair HCMV primary infection, as is seen with the CCR5 Δ32 mutation and HIV [17]. HCMV seronegative individuals have increased longevity, possibly linked with reduced clonal expansion of CD8 T cells and a larger reservoir of circulating naive T cells [18, 19] so early childhood primary infection with HCMV in sub-Saharan Africa may have profound effects. There is evidence linking early HCMV infections in sub-Saharan Africa with impaired physical and mental development [3], analogous to the known developmental CNS defects (hearing loss, mental retardation, cerebral palsy, seizures, chorioretinitis) caused by congenital HCMV infection [20, 21].

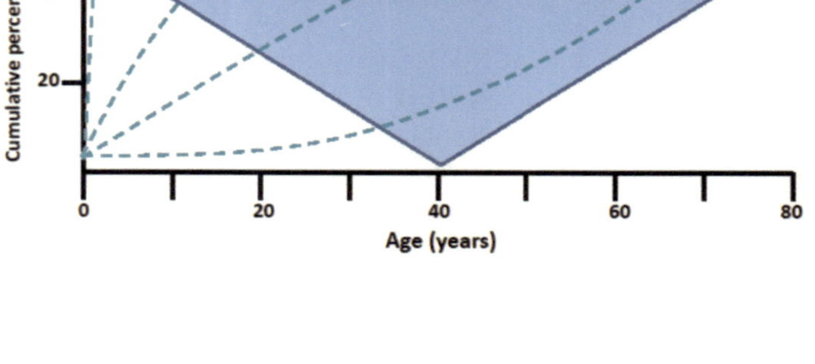

Figure 1. Model for the cumulative prevalence of primary HCMV seroconversion by age with respect to socioeconomic status (SES) groups.

Country (City)	HCMV IgG seroprevalence*	Study population	N=	Assay	Reference
HIV- Adults	**79.3%**				
Nigeria (Ibadan)	55.0%	Adult healthy blood donors	110	Compliment fixation	[22]
Mali (Bamako)	58.0%	Adult healthy HIV-ve blood donors	100	ELISA (Platelia® Sanofi Pasteur)	[23]
Tanzania (Dar Es Salaam)	66.9%	Adult inpatients with STDs (HIV-ve)	158	Passive latex agglutination (CMV-scan card)	[24]
Ghana (Accra)	77.6%	Adult healthy HIV-ve blood donors	3275	ELISA IgG; Diamedix Corporation, USA	[25]
Burkina Faso (Bobo Dioulasso)	82.0%	Adult healthy HIV-ve blood donors	28	ELISA (Platelia® Sanofi Pasteur)	[26]
Ghana (Kumasi)	94.3%	Health Blood Donors	112	Platella TM CMV IgG (Bio-Rad)	[27]
Somalia (Mogadishu)	96%	Healthy adult makes	102	unspecified	[28]
Somalia (Mogadishu)	96%	Adult males attending STD clinic	101	unspecified	[28]
Kenya (Nairobi)	97.0%	Adult healthy blood donors (1.3% HIV+)	400	unspecified	[29]
HIV+ Adults	**80.0%**				
Mali (Bamako)	71.0%	HIV+ Adults	100	ELISA (Platelia® Sanofi Pasteur)	[23]
Tanzania (Dar Es Salaam)	72.3%	Adult inpatients with STDs (HIV+ve)	65	Passive latex agglutination (CMV-scan card)	[24]
Ghana (Kumasi)	92.7%	Asymptomatic HIV+ Adults	55	Platella TM CMV IgG (Bio-Rad)	[27]
Botswana (Gaborone)	96.3%	Asymptomatic HIV+ Adults	43		[30]
AIDS Patients	**81.9%**				
Ghana (Accra)	59.2%	AIDS patients	250	ELISA IgG; Diamedix Corporation, USA	[25]
Mali (Bamako)	89.0%	AIDS patients	100	ELISA (Platelia® Sanofi Pasteur)	[23]
Tanzania (Dar Es Salaam)	90.7%	AIDS patients	43	Passive latex agglutination (CMV-scan card)	[24]
Ghana (Kumasi)	98.3%	AIDS patients	239	Platella TM CMV IgG (Bio-Rad)	[27]
Burkina Faso (Bobo Dioulasso)	100%	AIDS patients	36	ELISA (Platelia® Sanofi Pasteur)	[26]
Pregnant Women	**86.3%**				
Tanzania (Dar Es Salaam)	60.6%	HIV-ve pregnant women	127	Passive latex agglutination (CMV-scan card)	[24]
Tanzania (Dar Es Salaam)	85.7%	HIV+ve pregnant women	14	Passive latex agglutination (CMV-scan card)	[24]
Benin (Cotonou)	97.2%	Pregnant women	211	ETI-CYTOK-G PLUS ELISA (DiaSorin)	[31]
Nigeria (Ibadan)	100%	Pregnant (some not pregnant) women	80	peroxidase enzyme-labelled antigen (ELA)	[5]
South Africa (Johannesburg)	86.4%	Pregnant Women	2160	ELISA (M A Bioproducts, Virginia)	[32]
Children	**88.4%**				
Cameroon (Kumba City)	88.5%	Healthy Children 4-6 years	~100	ELISA (unspecified)	[33]
Cameroon (Kumba City)	98.0%	Healthy Children 11-14 years	~100	ELISA (unspecified)	[33]
Gambia (Banjul)	86.4%	Healthy Children 12 months	178	Immunofluoruescence?	[4]
Mozambique (SE Transvaal)	88.0%	Refugee Children under 5yrs	~100	ELISA (unspecified)	[34]
Mozambique (SE Transvaal)	96.4%	Refugee Children under 11 years	~100	ELISA (unspecified)	[34]
Nigeria (Ibadan)	100%	Newborn Infants	21	peroxidase enzyme-labelled antigen (ELA)	[5]
Zambia (Lusaka)	83%	Healthy 18-month old infants	460	ETI-CYTOK-G PLUS ELISA (DiaSorin)	[3]
Kenya (Nairobi)	100%	HIV-1 infected street children	71	ELISA kit (Murex)	[35]
Tuberculosis studies	**83.0%**				
Nigeria (Ibadan)	50.6%	Non-TB	89	Compliment fixation	[22]
Nigeria (Ibadan)	87.6%	Tuberculosis Patients	161	Compliment fixation	[22]
Burkina Faso (Bobo Dioulasso)	95.0%	TB+ HIV+ve	40	ELISA (Platelia® Sanofi Pasteur)	[26]
Burkina Faso (Bobo Dioulasso)	96.5%	Tuberculosis Patients	80	ELISA (Platelia® Sanofi Pasteur)	[26]
Burkina Faso (Bobo Dioulasso)	97.5%	TB+ HIV-ve	40	ELISA (Platelia® Sanofi Pasteur)	[26]
Other	**95.9%**				
Eritrea (various locations)	94.8%	Various	439	ELISA (unspecified)	[36]
Burundi (Bujumbura)	99.0%	Ophthalmic patients	154	ELISA Enzygnost CMV (Abbott Laboratories, Chicago, IL, USA	[37]

Table 1. Comparison of HCMV seroprevalence in different countries * Percentages in bold are the averages within each group, weighted by study size.

1.1.2. Molecular epidemiology

HCMV has a large genome, predicted to encode at least 165 proteins. This includes hypervariable segments [38-41] containing genes which encode membrane-bound glycoproteins. These are embedded in the virion envelope or presented on the surface of infected cells, making them candidate targets for the host immune response. Most published studies of polymorphisms in these glycoproteins have concentrated on possible associations with and clinical disease or cellular tropism. No compelling connections have been reported in the literature to date, but much of the sequence data is from isolates from Europe, North America and Japan.

There is little information regarding HCMV genotypes in Africa. In an early study investigating geographic differences in the frequency of certain HCMV genotypes from immunocompromised patients, they found that the distribution differed between Zimbabwe, Italy and California [42]. This study was limited to UL55 (virion surface glycoprotein gB: involved in cell entry and signaling)[43] which is relatively conserved between strains [40] and not linked with more variable glycoproteins [44]. A study of HCMV strains from 19 Malawian Kaposi's sarcoma (KS) patients and 58 of their first-degree relatives detected HCMV readily in mouth rinse and urine specimens [45]. Two hypervariable glycoprotein genes were sequenced: gO (UL74) and gN (UL73) involved in promoting focal spread [46, 47] and virion morphogenesis and possible latency associated functions respectively [48, 49]. Studies from Zambia segregate variants of these two glycoproteins into eight linked groups [50, 51]. These studies and others from Africa have found evidence of co-infections with multiple HCMV strains [50, 52] and no evidence for geographic separation. This data contrasts with other herpesviruses such as HHV-6 [53] and KSHV [54]. The high prevalence of co-infections with multiple strains, in a broad range of patients, complicates genotyping studies and attempts to identify disease links with specific glycoprotein genotypes. New techniques combining PCR amplification with RFLP digestion could improve analysis of multiple strains and recombinants in pathological samples [55].

2. HCMV infections and HIV in Sub-Saharan Africa

2.1. General considerations

sub-Saharan Africa is at the epicentre of the HIV pandemic, with 1,900,000 new infections (18.9% children ≤ 14yrs of age) in 2010, and a total of 23.2 million people (13.4% children ≤ 14yrs of age) living with HIV. Progress is slow but new infections are down 16% on 2001, and HIV prevalence has declined in some sub-Saharan African countries. With the roll out of antiretroviral therapy (ART), the numbers of people dying from HIV is also down (30% decrease between 2004 and 2010) [56]. HCMV is an apex opportunistic pathogen, linked with HIV disease progression [57-59], so the HIV pandemic combined with over 80% of primary HCMV infections occurring during infancy, creates a unique environment. Active HCMV infections are common and present as complex co-infections with other viral, bacterial and fungal infections [60, 61]. A broader awareness of the frequency of co-infections and the complex interplay between different pathogens is needed.

http://dx.doi.org/10.5772/54907

2.2. Disease presentations and co-morbidity

The most common presentation of HCMV infection in HIV-infected patients is HCMV pneumonia, where co-infection with other respiratory pathogens such a tuberculosis and *Pneumocystis jirovecci,* is almost ubiquitous [50, 60]. HCMV is an important HIV co-infection, also linked with a range diseases including meningitis [62], encephalitis [63], psychological disorders [64], malaria [65], various dermatological conditions [66, 67] and those affecting mucosal epithelia [68, 69], hypoadrenalism [70], adrenalitis [71], gastritis [72, 73] and other herpesvirus infections [74]. There has been a huge (possibly disproportionate) focus on HCMV as a cause of HIV-associated retinitis. Globally it has been estimated that 5-25% of AIDS patients will suffer from HCMV retinitis in their lifetime [75] leading to an 'epidemic of blindness' [76]. Whilst the cohorts and diagnostic methods vary in different studies, HIV-associated HCMV retinitis is less common in sub-Saharan Africa than elsewhere, seen in just 0-8.5% of adult AIDS patients with ophthalmic conditions [77-83].

2.3. HCMV as a cause of death

It is unclear how much active HCMV infection is contributing to mortality in HIV infected people. One way to address this question is to measure mortality as a primary outcome. For example: a large longitudinal study of HIV infected miners in South Africa associated HCMV viraemia with a three-fold increase in mortality after just 11 months. The affect was weakened when controlling for CD4 T-cell count, WHO stage and HIV viral load– all conditions predictive of mortality [84]. A study of HIV-infected and -exposed Kenyan children found a strong correlation between HIV-1 and HCMV viral loads. Adjusting for maternal immunosuppression and HIV-1 viral load, HCMV viraemia during pregnancy was linked with high risk of death for mothers and infants in the 2 years following delivery [85]. It is difficult to prove that HCMV viraemia is not simply a bystander and is actually involved in pathology. This requires post mortem studies, which are difficult due to cultural factors [86]. Paediatric post mortem studies from sub-Saharan Africa identify HCMV as a common cause of death [87, 88], especially in HIV infected patients [89-91]. There is a need for new post-mortem data, from both prospective studies and routine cases, to better inform on the prevalence of active HCMV as a cause of death, and in particular, to calibrate HCMV viral loads pre-mortem with histopathological evidence of active HCMV infection post-mortem [92].

3. HCMV pneumonia in HIV infected children

Pneumonia is the most common cause of death in children <5 yrs of age globally, accounting for 18% of all deaths [93]. In sub-Saharan Africa, pneumonia is the leading cause of death in HIV-infected and -exposed children [94-97]. Across the region antibiotics are cheap and widely available, yet pneumonia is still a major cause of paediatric mortality. This is likely in part due to antibiotic resistance [98], but also several viral pathogens cause lower respiratory tract infections and remain undiagnosed and untreated.

HCMV pneumonia is very common in HIV-infected and –exposed in sub-Saharan Africa [99, 100] and is associated with rapid progression of HIV disease [101] and death [102-104]. A seminal post mortem study in 264 Zambian children who died of respiratory disease identified classical HCMV inclusions in the lung tissue of up to 22% of HIV-infected cases [60], and then follow-up molecular work found high loads of HCMV were virtually ubiquitous in the lung tissue of HIV-infected paediatric respiratory deaths [50]. HCMV pneumonia is virtually impossible to distinguish clinically from *Pneumocystis jirovecci* pneumonia and co-infections with both *Pneumocystis jirovecci* and tuberculosis are common in HIV-infected and -exposed infants [60, 61, 105]. In South Africa, HCMV pneumonia was more common than *Pneumocystis jirovecci* pneumonia and other viral pneumonias in HIV-infected children [106], and was histologically confirmed in 72% of HIV-infected and ventilated infant mortalities with severe pneumonia. The authors recommend empiric use of ganciclovir or other anti-HCMV drugs in HIV-infected children with severe pneumonia who are not responding to co-trimoxazole [107].

4. HCMV Congenital Infection in sub-Saharan Africa

Congenital HCMV is generally defined by the detection of viral DNA and/or IgM antibody in infant sera within the first 3 weeks post-partum [108]. It is a damaging infection initiated by either primary or reactivated infection in the mother during pregnancy, although congenital HCMV infections transmitted from mothers with pre-existing immunity can be less severe [109]. Congenital HCMV is the major viral cause of mental and physical disability in children, infecting 0.2-2.2% of newborns [110, 111]. Around 7-11% of infected foetuses are then born with symptoms [112, 113], with a neonatal mortality rate of 20-30% [114, 115]. Of those congenitally infected (both symptomatic and asymptomatic), up to 28% will develop late sequelae [116]. Symptoms include growth retardation, hepatosplenomegaly, jaundice, pneumonia, gastrointestinal, and neurological disease such as sensorineural hearing loss, mental retardation, chorioretinitis, seizures [117] and cerebral palsy [118].

Congenital HCMV infection was considered rare in populations with high adult seroprevalence [33]. A study of 2032 newborn infants in the Ivory Coast cultured HCMV from urine and showed congenital HCMV infection in 1.4% of all births [119]. In sub-Saharan Africa, congenital HCMV largely reflects maternal reactivations or re-infections, which may not result in severe disease in the child [109]. However, a few studies from the region suggest congenital HCMV maybe a significant cause of morbidity and mortality. A study from Zambia associated HCMV antibody titres above 1:1024 with still births [120]. HCMV IgM antibodies were detected in 24% of 99 newborn babies who were jaundiced, died within a few days of birth or showed gross congenital abnormalities [121]. Cervical shedding of HCMV is very common in HIV-infected women, and is readily detected in amniotic fluid collected at C-section [122, 123]. A Gambian study found the prevalence of congenital CMV among healthy neonates was 5.4%, at least 2-fold higher than reported in industrialized countries. Congenitally infected children were more often first born babies, more frequently born in crowded compounds and active placental malaria was more prevalent. During the first year of follow up, mothers of congenitally infected children reported more health complaints for their child [124]. Recently a study from Zambia has shown that HCMV seroprevalence in 18 month old infants is linked with impaired growth and mental development [3]. There is a need for more prospective studies to investigate the clinical significance of congenital HCMV infections in sub-Saharan Africa.

5. HCMV diagnosis and treatment in Sub-Saharan Africa

One of the greatest challenges for HCMV diagnosis in this region is to differentiate clinically active from sub-clinical infection. Serological tests for HCMV IgM are useful for diagnosing primary infections in infants, particularly congenital infections in neonates, but the majority of the disease burden is caused by re-activation or re-infections in immunocompromised patients. Detection of the virus itself was traditionally achieved using culture-based methods. These are time-consuming and require well-trained staff and a well-serviced diagnostic laboratory. Moreover, HCMV culture is not very sensitive. For these reasons, quantitative DNA-based molecular diagnostics are now commonly used to detect active HCMV infections. The required infrastructure is becoming commonly available at tertiary and secondary referral centres across sub-Saharan Africa, often donated by international research projects. However low level HCMV reactivations are common in a wide range of patients, linked with reduced immune surveillance due to other infections, illness or malnutrition.

Most studies of HCMV viral loads with respect to disease outcomes are in the transplant field, where viral loads within the range of 10^4 to 10^6 copies/ml whole blood have been suggested to be indicative of active disease, depending on the specific patient group [125]. An autopsy study found that a cut off of 10^4 copies/ml whole blood, gave a specificity and positive predictive value of 100% for HCMV disease, making the commercial assay used (COBAS AMPLICOR CMV Monitor test - Roche) better for 'ruling in', than 'ruling out' [126]. There is a need for prospective studies in sub-Saharan Africa to monitor HCMV viral loads in patients with HIV-associated pneumonia, and infants with congenital HCMV infection, the two major HCMV disease groups in the region – although there are also transplant recipients in sub-Saharan Africa [127]. HCMV is shed in high loads in both urine and saliva (non-invasive specimens ideal for low income settings) and detection of virus DNA in these specimens should be evaluated versus viraemia, as potentially useful markers of active disease.

Several drugs are licensed for the treatment of HCMV infections, although they are expensive and broadly unavailable in sub-Saharan Africa. At some tertiary referral centres in South Africa, intravenous ganciclovir is used to treat HCMV pneumonia in HIV-infected and -exposed children failing antibiotic or anti-mycobacterial therapy. Decisions are largely consultant led but two descriptive studies have reported dramatic reductions in mortality due to ganciclovir [106, 107]. Readers are advised to look up the latest guidelines on treatment of HCMV and to check the correct doses, side effects and dosing schedules. In South African centres, PCR or culture-proven HCMV disease is typically treated with 5mg/kg intravenously every 12hrs for 14-21 days, and then daily maintenance therapy at 5mg/kg [94]. But there is an urgent need for further descriptive studies to identify patients for treatment. Randomized controlled clinical trials are needed to evaluate safety and efficacy.

The introduction of expensive antiviral treatments in low income settings is always problematic; Ethics review boards may state that it is unethical to trial antiviral drugs which are unaffordable and inaccessible to the majority of the affected patients. The path to new treatments has to start somewhere, and as scientists we favour evidence as the basis for action. The case of CD4 testing and antiretroviral therapy has proven that resources can be mobilized from a range of stake holders, including governments, NGOs and private enterprise [128-130]. A second ethical dilemma is that if the drug is being used successfully in South Africa to treat HIV-associated HCMV pneumonia, is it ethical for Ganciclovir trials to administer placebos? When answering such ethical questions we should note that HCMV affects a broad range of patient groups across sub-Saharan Africa, including congenitally infected neonates, HIV infected infants, children and adults causing pneumonia, specific organ disease (eg. retinitis, encephalitis, gastritis) and disseminated infection. Furthermore, malnutrition and co-infection with other common pathogens (Malaria, Tuberculosis, *Pneumocystis Jirovecci* etc..) are prevalent. For this diverse patient group, the evidence base for the optimal dose, duration and route of administration is poor [131].

6. Effect of HCMV on vaccine efficacy and immune senescence in Sub-Saharan Africa

Infant vaccination programmes are a central component of national paediatric disease prevention strategies in sub-Saharan Africa [132], but they are less effective than equivalent programmes in high income populations. For example: The efficacy of live attenuated measles virus vaccine in Europe and North America is over 90% [133-135] whereas in West Africa it is below 70% [136-138]. This could be partly due to the higher infectious disease burden in sub-Saharan Africa, which may affect antibody [139, 140] and cytokine [141] responses to vaccination, and also reduced vaccine performance in HIV-infected children [132]. With 3.1 million children living with HIV/AIDS across the region [56], vaccine safety and efficacy must be independently assessed in this significant and vulnerable patient group. HIV-infected children can generally seroconvert in response to both live-attenuated and inactivated/subunit vaccines, but the immune response is generally weaker with lower antibody levels and seroprotection rates in HIV-infected children [142-144]. The weaker immune response in HIV-infected children could be due to defective antigen presentation, defective B-cell priming or impaired differentiation into memory cells, impaired primary response due to low CD4, loss of protective antibodies or loss of immunological memory of T and B cells after priming [143].

Most HIV-infected children in sub-Saharan Africa will also be infected with HCMV, which encodes over thirty genes with potential immunomodulatory functions. These genes may affect classical and non-classical major histocompatibility complex (MHC) protein function, leukocyte migration and activation, cytokine responses and host cell susceptibility to apoptosis [43]. HCMV can infect and initiate gene expression in an extraordinarily broad range of cell

http://dx.doi.org/10.5772/54907

types, although IE gene transcripts have not been detected in T- or B-lymphocytes [145, 146]. Despite this, HCMV influences cell-mediated immunity. T-cell populations in HCMV-infected infants in the Gambia showed higher levels of differentiation [147, 148] and similar HCMV-induced differentiation in elderly non-African populations is associated with depleted naive T-cell populations and impaired vaccine responses [149]. HCMV infection is also associated with a decline in naive T cells and impaired T-cell reconstitution in HIV infected adults initiating HAART [150]. But naive T-cell populations appear unaffected by HCMV infection in African children, and infection was not linked with impaired T-cell responses to measles virus vaccination [151], with HCMV activated T-helpers possibly improving measles antibody response [152]. A study in older African children, found that HIV-negative Malawian teenagers had a lower percentage of naïve T cells, higher memory T and higher CD28- memory T-cells, compared to age-matched UK teenagers. Whilst all of the adolescents tested in Malawi were seropositive for HCMV, seroprevalence was just 36% in the UK group, and was associated with a reduced percentage of naïve T cells and an increased percentage of CD28- memory T cells in the periphery [153].

Whilst more evidence is required, these studies suggest early infant infection with HCMV, and maybe a general higher burden of infectious disease, contribute to a more rapid ageing of the immune system in sub-Saharan Africa. Whilst access to anti-HCMV drugs would likely significantly reduce morbidity and mortality in acute HCMV infections, such as congenitally infected infants or HIV/AIDS patients with pneumonia or disseminated HCMV, the implications of a successful HCMV vaccine have potentially far-reaching benefits across the region. Future studies evaluating vaccine efficacy in sub-Saharan Africa should stratify by HCMV serostatus, and where facilities permit, include work on HCMV genotypes and flow cytometric analysis to further characterise the effect of infant HCMV infection on immunity.

7. Summary

In sub-Saharan Africa, HCMV infection is endemic in young infants where it is linked with impaired physical and mental development [3], giving the infection a unique epidemiology across the region, with a potentially broad-reaching impact on the health of southern African populations. Studies conducted in sub-Saharan Africa and elsewhere, have shown that HCMV is a serious cause or morbidity and mortality, in both immunocompromised groups and congenitally infected children. In a region where 23.2 million people are living with HIV and most of the population are infected with HCMV in infancy [124], more prospective studies are required to better characterise the impact of HCMV in sub-Saharan Africa. This will lay the foundations for future clinical trials of anti-HCMV drugs in patient sub-sets in whom there is strong evidence that they might be effective. Drugs such as ganciclovir are already used in South Africa as life-saving treatment for HIV-infected children with severe pneumonia that is not responsive to antibiotic or anti-mycobacterial therapy. Furthermore, the clinical impact and importance of HCMV infections in sub-Saharan Africa may increase over the next decade for several reasons: Wider access to ART is resulting in increasing numbers of older HIV infected patients; Cancer incidence is forecast to increase by 32% across sub-Saharan Africa between 2010 and 2020 [154]; The number of transplant recipients is also set to increase, as the capacity of tertiary care centres develops and improves.

Acknowledgements

This work was supported by the European Commission (grant ADAT-number SANTE/ 2006/129-131). AZ is grant holder and MB study coordinator. AZ and MB are supported by the European and Developing Countries Clinical Trials Partnership (EDCTP grants REMOX, PANACEA and TB-NEAT), Netherlands; UK Medical Research Council (MRC); UBS Optimus Foundation, Switzerland; University College London Hospitals Comprehensive Biomedical Research Centre (UCLH-CBRC); and the UCLH National Health Service (NHS) Foundation Trust. KM is supported by the Commonwealth Scholarship Commission, U.K.

Author details

Matthew Bates[1,2*], Kunda Musonda[1,2,3] and Alimuddin Zumla[2]

*Address all correspondence to: matthew.bates@ucl.ac.uk

1 UNZA-UCLMS Research and Training Programme and HerpeZ, University of Zambia School of Medicine/University Teaching Hospital, Lusaka, Zambia

2 University College London (UCL) Medical School, Department of Infection, Centre for Infectious Diseases and International Health, Royal Free Hospital, London, UK

3 London School of Hygiene and Tropical Medicine (LSHTM), Department of Infectious Tropical Diseases, Pathogen Molecular Biology Unit, London, UK

References

[1] Booth JC, Hannington G, Bakir TM, Stern H, Kangro H, Griffiths PD, et al. Comparison of enzyme-linked immunosorbent assay, radioimmunoassay, complement fixation, anticomplement immunofluorescence and passive haemagglutination techniques for detecting cytomegalovirus IgG antibody. J Clin Pathol. 1982 Dec;35(12):1345-8.

[2] Booth JC, Kangro HO, Liu KM, el Mohandes L, Tryhorn YS. Discordant results obtained on testing sera from immunocompromised patients for cytomegalovirus IgG by enzyme-linked immunosorbent assay and radioimmunoassay. J Virol Methods. 1989 Oct;26(1):77-89.

[3] Gompels UA, Larke N, Sanz-Ramos M, Bates M, Musonda K, Manno D, et al. Human cytomegalovirus infant infection adversely affects growth and development in maternally HIV-exposed and unexposed infants in Zambia. Clin Infect Dis. 2012 Feb 1;54(3):434-42.

[4] Bello C, Whittle H. Cytomegalovirus infection in Gambian mothers and their babies. J Clin Pathol. 1991 May;44(5):366-9.

[5] Williams JO, Fagbami AH, Omilabu SA. Cytomegalovirus antibodies in Nigeria. Trans R Soc Trop Med Hyg. 1989 Mar-Apr;83(2):260.

[6] Staras SA, Dollard SC, Radford KW, Flanders WD, Pass RF, Cannon MJ. Seroprevalence of cytomegalovirus infection in the United States, 1988-1994. Clin Infect Dis. 2006 Nov 1;43(9):1143-51.

[7] Cannon MJ, Schmid DS, Hyde TB. Review of cytomegalovirus seroprevalence and demographic characteristics associated with infection. Rev Med Virol. 2010 Jul;20(4):202-13.

[8] Tookey PA, Ades AE, Peckham CS. Cytomegalovirus prevalence in pregnant women: the influence of parity. Arch Dis Child. 1992 Jul;67(7 Spec No):779-83.

[9] Green MS, Cohen D, Slepon R, Robin G, Wiener M. Ethnic and gender differences in the prevalence of anti-cytomegalovirus antibodies among young adults in Israel. Int J Epidemiol. 1993 Aug;22(4):720-3.

[10] Ahlfors K, Ivarsson SA, Johnsson T, Svanberg L. Primary and secondary maternal cytomegalovirus infections and their relation to congenital infection. Analysis of maternal sera. Acta Paediatr Scand. 1982 Jan;71(1):109-13.

[11] Numazaki K, Fujikawa T, Chiba S. Relationship between seropositivity of husbands and primary cytomegalovirus infection during pregnancy. J Infect Chemother. 2000 Jun;6(2):104-6.

[12] Bello CS. Transmission of cytomegalovirus in the Gambia. West Afr J Med. 1992 Apr-Jun;11(2):140-5.

[13] Butler LM, Neilands TB, Mosam A, Mzolo S, Martin JN. A population-based study of how children are exposed to saliva in KwaZulu-Natal Province, South Africa: implications for the spread of saliva-borne pathogens to children. Trop Med Int Health. 2010 Apr;15(4):442-53.

[14] Jim WT, Shu CH, Chiu NC, Chang JH, Hung HY, Peng CC, et al. High cytomegalovirus load and prolonged virus excretion in breast milk increase risk for viral acquisition by very low birth weight infants. Pediatr Infect Dis J. 2009 Oct;28(10):891-4.

[15] Kerrey BT, Morrow A, Geraghty S, Huey N, Sapsford A, Schleiss MR. Breast milk as a source for acquisition of cytomegalovirus (HCMV) in a

premature infant with sepsis syndrome: detection by real-time PCR. J Clin Virol. 2006 Mar;35(3):313-6.

[16] Oginni FO, Alao OO, Mamman A, Araoye MO, Joseph E. Effect of Demographic Variables on Cytomegalovirus Antibody Seropositivity among Prospective Blood Donors in Jos, Nigeria. Niger Postgrad Med J. 2009 Mar; 16(1):21-4.

[17] Blanpain C, Libert F, Vassart G, Parmentier M. CCR5 and HIV infection. Receptors Channels. 2002;8(1):19-31.

[18] Hadrup SR, Strindhall J, Kollgaard T, Seremet T, Johansson B, Pawelec G, et al. Longitudinal studies of clonally expanded CD8 T cells reveal a repertoire shrinkage predicting mortality and an increased number of dysfunctional cytomegalovirus-specific T cells in the very elderly. J Immunol. 2006 Feb 15;176(4):2645-53.

[19] Khan N, Shariff N, Cobbold M, Bruton R, Ainsworth JA, Sinclair AJ, et al. Cytomegalovirus seropositivity drives the CD8 T cell repertoire toward greater clonality in healthy elderly individuals. J Immunol. 2002 Aug 15;169(4):1984-92.

[20] Pass RF. Congenital cytomegalovirus infection and hearing loss. Herpes. 2005 Oct;12(2):50-5.

[21] Pass RF, Fowler KB, Boppana SB, Britt WJ, Stagno S. Congenital cytomegalovirus infection following first trimester maternal infection: symptoms at birth and outcome. J Clin Virol. 2006 Feb;35(2):216-20.

[22] Olaleye OD, Omilabu SA, Baba SS. Cytomegalovirus infection among tuberculosis patients in a chest hospital in Nigeria. Comp Immunol Microbiol Infect Dis. 1990;13(2):101-6.

[23] Maiga, II, Tounkara A, Coulibaly G, Kouriba B. [Seroprevalence of the human cytomegalovirus among blood donors and AIDS patients in Bamako]. Sante. 2003 Apr-Jun;13(2):117-9.

[24] Mhalu F, Haukenes G. Prevalence of cytomegalovirus antibody in pregnant women, AIDS patients and STD patients in Dar es Salaam. AIDS. 1990 Dec;4(12):1294-5.

[25] Adjei AA, Armah HB, Gbagbo F, Boamah I, Adu-Gyamfi C, Asare I. Seroprevalence of HHV-8, CMV, and EBV among the general population in Ghana, West Africa. BMC Infect Dis. 2008;8:111.

[26] Ledru E, Diagbouga S, Ledru S, Cauchoix B, Yameogo M, Chami D, et al. A study of Toxoplasma and Cytomegalovirus serology in tuberculosis and in HIV-infected patients in Burkina Faso. Acta Trop. 1995 May;59(2): 149-54.

[27] Compston LI, Li C, Sarkodie F, Owusu-Ofori S, Opare-Sem O, Allain JP. Prevalence of persistent and latent viruses in untreated patients infected with HIV-1 from Ghana, West Africa. J Med Virol. 2009 Nov;81(11):1860-8.

[28] Ismail SO, Ahmed HJ, Grillner L, Hederstedt B, Issa A, Bygdeman SM. Sexually transmitted diseases in men in Mogadishu, Somalia. Int J STD AIDS. 1990 Mar;1(2):102-6.

[29] Njeru DG, Mwanda WO, Kitonyi GW, Njagi EC. Prevalence of cytomegalovirus antibodies in blood donors at the National Blood Transfusion Centre, Nairobi. East Afr Med J. 2009 Dec;86(12 Suppl):S58-61.

[30] Wester CW, Bussmann H, Moyo S, Avalos A, Gaolathe T, Ndwapi N, et al. Serological evidence of HIV-associated infection among HIV-1-infected adults in Botswana. Clin Infect Dis. 2006 Dec 15;43(12):1612-5.

[31] Rodier MH, Berthonneau J, Bourgoin A, Giraudeau G, Agius G, Burucoa C, et al. Seroprevalences of Toxoplasma, malaria, rubella, cytomegalovirus, HIV and treponemal infections among pregnant women in Cotonou, Republic of Benin. Acta Trop. 1995 Aug;59(4):271-7.

[32] Schoub BD, Johnson S, McAnerney JM, Blackburn NK, Guidozzi F, Ballot D, et al. Is antenatal screening for rubella and cytomegalovirus justified? S Afr Med J. 1993 Feb;83(2):108-10.

[33] Stroffolini T, Ngatchu T, Chiaramonte M, Giammanco A, Maggio M, Sarzana A, et al. Prevalence of cytomegalovirus seropositivity in an urban childhood population in Cameroon. New Microbiol. 1993 Jan;16(1):83-5.

[34] Bos P, Steele AD, Peenze I, Aspinall S. Sero-prevalence to hepatitis B and C virus infection in refugees from Mozambique in southern Africa. East Afr Med J. 1995 Feb;72(2):113-5.

[35] Chakraborty R, Rees G, Bourboulia D, Cross AM, Dixon JR, D'Agostino A, et al. Viral coinfections among African children infected with human immunodeficiency virus type 1. Clin Infect Dis. 2003 Apr 1;36(7):922-4.

[36] Ghebrekidan H, Ruden U, Cox S, Wahren B, Grandien M. Prevalence of herpes simplex virus types 1 and 2, cytomegalovirus, and varicella-zoster virus infections in Eritrea. J Clin Virol. 1999 Jan;12(1):53-64.

[37] Cochereau I, Mlika-Cabanne N, Godinaud P, Niyongabo T, Poste B, Ngayiragije A, et al. AIDS related eye disease in Burundi, Africa. Br J Ophthalmol. 1999 Mar;83(3):339-42.

[38] Murphy E, Yu D, Grimwood J, Schmutz J, Dickson M, Jarvis MA, et al. Coding potential of laboratory and clinical strains of human cytomegalovirus. Proc Natl Acad Sci U S A. 2003 Dec 9;100(25):14976-81.

[39] Davison AJ, Dolan A, Akter P, Addison C, Dargan DJ, Alcendor DJ, et al. The human cytomegalovirus genome revisited: comparison with the chimpanzee cytomegalovirus genome. J Gen Virol. 2003 Jan;84(Pt 1):17-28.

[40] Dolan A, Cunningham C, Hector RD, Hassan-Walker AF, Lee L, Addison C, et al. Genetic content of wild-type human cytomegalovirus. J Gen Virol. 2004 May;85(Pt 5):1301-12.

[41] Qi Y, Mao ZQ, Ruan Q, He R, Ma YP, Sun ZR, et al. Human cytomegalovirus (HCMV) UL139 open reading frame: Sequence variants are clustered into three major genotypes. J Med Virol. 2006 Apr;78(4):517-22.

[42] Zipeto D, Hong C, Gerna G, Zavattoni M, Katzenstein D, Merigan TC, et al. Geographic and demographic differences in the frequency of human cytomegalovirus gB genotypes 1-4 in immunocompromised patients. AIDS Res Hum Retroviruses. 1998 Apr 10;14(6):533-6.

[43] Mocarski ES, Jr; Shenk, T; Pass, R.F. Cytomegaloviruses. In: D.M Knipe PMHea, editor. Fields Virology. 5 ed. Philidelphia: Lippincot, Williams and Wilkins; 2007. p. 2701-72.

[44] Rasmussen L, Geissler A, Winters M. Inter- and intragenic variations complicate the molecular epidemiology of human cytomegalovirus. J Infect Dis. 2003 Mar 1;187(5):809-19.

[45] Beyari MM, Hodgson TA, Kondowe W, Molyneux EM, Scully C, Porter SR, et al. Inter- and intra-person cytomegalovirus infection in Malawian families. J Med Virol. 2005 Apr;75(4):575-82.

[46] Jiang XJ, Adler B, Sampaio KL, Digel M, Jahn G, Ettischer N, et al. UL74 of human cytomegalovirus contributes to virus release by promoting secondary envelopment of virions. J Virol. 2008 Jan 9.

[47] Jiang XJ, Sampaio KL, Ettischer N, Stierhof YD, Jahn G, Kropff B, et al. UL74 of human cytomegalovirus reduces the inhibitory effect of gH-specific and gB-specific antibodies. Arch Virol. 2011 Dec;156(12):2145-55.

[48] Mach M, Osinski K, Kropff B, Schloetzer-Schrehardt U, Krzyzaniak M, Britt W. The carboxy-terminal domain of glycoprotein N of human cytomegalovirus is required for virion morphogenesis. J Virol. 2007 May;81(10):5212-24.

[49] Pignatelli S, Dal Monte P, Rossini G, Camozzi D, Toscano V, Conte R, et al. Latency-associated human cytomegalovirus glycoprotein N genotypes in monocytes from healthy blood donors. Transfusion. 2006 Oct;46(10):1754-62.

[50] Bates M, Monze M, Bima H, Kapambwe M, Kasolo FC, Gompels UA. High human cytomegalovirus loads and diverse linked variable genotypes in both HIV-1 infected and exposed, but uninfected, children in Africa. Virology. 2008 Dec 5;382(1):28-36.

[51] Mattick C, Dewin D, Polley S, Sevilla-Reyes E, Pignatelli S, Rawlinson W, et al. Linkage of human cytomegalovirus glycoprotein gO variant groups identified from worldwide clinical isolates with gN genotypes, implications for disease associations and evidence for N-terminal sites of positive selection. Virology. 2004 Jan 20;318(2):582-97.

[52] Bradley AJ, Kovacs IJ, Gatherer D, Dargan DJ, Alkharsah KR, Chan PK, et al. Genotypic analysis of two hypervariable human cytomegalovirus genes. J Med Virol. 2008 Sep;80(9):1615-23.

[53] Bates M, Monze M, Bima H, Kapambwe M, Clark D, Kasolo FC, et al. Predominant human herpesvirus 6 variant A infant infections in an HIV-1 endemic region of Sub-Saharan Africa. J Med Virol. 2009 May;81(5):779-89.

[54] Kasolo FC, Spinks J, Bima H, Bates M, Gompels UA. Diverse genotypes of Kaposi's sarcoma associated herpesvirus (KSHV) identified in infant blood infections in African childhood-KS and HIV/AIDS endemic region. J Med Virol. 2007 Oct;79(10):1555-61.

[55] Grosjean J, Hantz S, Cotin S, Baclet MC, Mengelle C, Trapes L, et al. Direct genotyping of cytomegalovirus envelope glycoproteins from toddler's saliva samples. J Clin Virol. 2009 Dec;46 Suppl 4:S43-8.

[56] WHO. Global HIV/AIDS response: epidemic update and health sector progress towards universal access: progress report 2011. WHO press; 2011.

[57] Kitchen BJ, Engler HD, Gill VJ, Marshall D, Steinberg SM, Pizzo PA, et al. Cytomegalovirus infection in children with human immunodeficiency virus infection. Pediatr Infect Dis J. 1997 Apr;16(4):358-63.

[58] Kovacs A, Schluchter M, Easley K, Demmler G, Shearer W, La Russa P, et al. Cytomegalovirus infection and HIV-1 disease progression in infants born to HIV-1-infected women. Pediatric Pulmonary and Cardiovascular Complications of Vertically Transmitted HIV Infection Study Group. N Engl J Med. 1999 Jul 8;341(2):77-84.

[59] Jeena PM, Coovadia HM, Bhagwanjee S. Prospective, controlled study of the outcome of human immunodeficiency virus-1 antibody-positive children admitted to an intensive care unit. Crit Care Med. 1996 Jun;24(6):963-7.

[60] Chintu C, Mudenda V, Lucas S, Nunn A, Lishimpi K, Maswahu D, et al. Lung diseases at necropsy in African children dying from respiratory illnesses: a descriptive necropsy study. Lancet. 2002 Sep 28;360(9338):985-90.

[61] Rennert WP, Kilner D, Hale M, Stevens G, Stevens W, Crewe-Brown H. Tuberculosis in children dying with HIV-related lung disease: clinical-pathological correlations. Int J Tuberc Lung Dis. 2002 Sep;6(9):806-13.

[62] Kelly MJ, Benjamin LA, Cartwright K, Ajdukiewicz KM, Cohen DB, Menyere M, et al. Epstein-barr virus coinfection in cerebrospinal fluid is

associated with increased mortality in Malawian adults with bacterial meningitis. J Infect Dis. 2011 Jan 1;205(1):106-10.

[63] Bell JE, Lowrie S, Koffi K, Honde M, Andoh J, De Cock KM, et al. The neuropathology of HIV-infected African children in Abidjan, Cote d'Ivoire. J Neuropathol Exp Neurol. 1997 Jun;56(6):686-92.

[64] Tedla Y, Shibre T, Ali O, Tadele G, Woldeamanuel Y, Asrat D, et al. Serum antibodies to Toxoplasma gondii and Herpesvidae family viruses in individuals with schizophrenia and bipolar disorder: a case-control study. Ethiop Med J. 2011 Jul;49(3):211-20.

[65] Harbarth S, Meyer M, Grau GE, Loutan L, Ricou B. Septic Shock due to Cytomegalovirus Infection in Acute Respiratory Distress Syndrome after Falciparum Malaria. J Travel Med. 1997 Sep 1;4(3):148-9.

[66] Grayson W. Recognition of Dual or Multiple Pathology in Skin Biopsies from Patients with HIV/AIDS. Patholog Res Int. 2011;2011:398546.

[67] Ramdial PK, Dlova NC, Sydney C. Cytomegalovirus neuritis in perineal ulcers. J Cutan Pathol. 2002 Aug;29(7):439-44.

[68] Grant HW. Patterns of presentation of human immunodeficiency virus type 1-infected children to the paediatric surgeon. J Pediatr Surg. 1999 Feb;34(2): 251-4.

[69] Contreras A, Falkler WA, Jr., Enwonwu CO, Idigbe EO, Savage KO, Afolabi MB, et al. Human Herpesviridae in acute necrotizing ulcerative gingivitis in children in Nigeria. Oral Microbiol Immunol. 1997 Oct;12(5): 259-65.

[70] Ekpebegh CO, Ogbera AO, Longo-Mbenza B, Blanco-Blanco E, Awotedu A, Oluboyo P. Basal cortisol levels and correlates of hypoadrenalism in patients with human immunodeficiency virus infection. Med Princ Pract. 2011;20(6):525-9.

[71] Unachukwu CN, Uchenna DI, Young EE. Endocrine and metabolic disorders associated with human immune deficiency virus infection. West Afr J Med. 2009 Jan;28(1):3-9.

[72] Harries A. Some clinical aspects of HIV infection in Africa. Afr Health. 1991 Jul;13(5):25-6.

[73] Cooke ML, Goddard EA, Brown RA. Endoscopy findings in HIV-infected children from Sub-Saharan Africa. J Trop Pediatr. 2009 Aug;55(4):238-43.

[74] Meer S, Altini M. Cytomegalovirus co-infection in AIDS-associated oral Kaposi's sarcoma. Adv Dent Res. 2006;19(1):96-8.

[75] Kestelyn PG, Cunningham ET, Jr. HIV/AIDS and blindness. Bull World Health Organ. 2001;79(3):208-13.

[76] Guex-Crosier Y, Telenti A. An epidemic of blindness: a consequence of improved HIV care? Bull World Health Organ. 2001;79(3):181.

[77] Pathai S, Gilbert C, Weiss HA, McNally M, Lawn SD. Differing spectrum of HIV-associated ophthalmic disease among patients starting antiretroviral therapy in India and South Africa. Trop Med Int Health. 2011 Mar;16(3): 356-9.

[78] Emina MO, Odjimogho SE. Ocular problems in HIV and AIDS patients in Nigeria. Optom Vis Sci. 2010 Dec;87(12):979-84.

[79] Nkomazana O, Tshitswana D. Ocular complications of HIV infection in sub-Sahara Africa. Curr HIV/AIDS Rep. 2008 Aug;5(3):120-5.

[80] Kestelyn P. The epidemiology of CMV retinitis in Africa. Ocul Immunol Inflamm. 1999 Dec;7(3-4):173-7.

[81] Beare NA, Kublin JG, Lewis DK, Schijffelen MJ, Peters RP, Joaki G, et al. Ocular disease in patients with tuberculosis and HIV presenting with fever in Africa. Br J Ophthalmol. 2002 Oct;86(10):1076-9.

[82] Balo KP, Amoussou YP, Bechetoille A, Mihluedo H, Djagnikpo PA, Akpandja SM, et al. [Cytomegalovirus retinitis and ocular complications in AIDS patients in Togo]. J Fr Ophtalmol. 1999 Dec;22(10):1042-6.

[83] Nirwoth JP, Hall AB, Lewallen S. Prevalence of cytomegalovirus retinitis in Tanzanians with low CD4 levels. Br J Ophthalmol. 2010 Apr;95(4):460-2.

[84] Fielding K, Koba A, Grant AD, Charalambous S, Day J, Spak C, et al. Cytomegalovirus viremia as a risk factor for mortality prior to antiretroviral therapy among HIV-infected gold miners in South Africa. PLoS One. 2011;6(10):e25571.

[85] Slyker JA, Lohman-Payne BL, John-Stewart GC, Maleche-Obimbo E, Emery S, Richardson B, et al. Acute cytomegalovirus infection in Kenyan HIV-infected infants. Aids. 2009 Oct 23;23(16):2173-81.

[86] Lishimpi K, Chintu C, Lucas S, Mudenda V, Kaluwaji J, Story A, et al. Necropsies in African children: consent dilemmas for parents and guardians. Arch Dis Child. 2001 Jun;84(6):463-7.

[87] Cox JA, Lukande RL, Lucas S, Nelson AM, Van Marck E, Colebunders R. Autopsy causes of death in HIV-positive individuals in Sub-Saharan Africa and correlation with clinical diagnoses. AIDS Rev. 2010 Oct-Dec;12(4):183-94.

[88] Martinson NA, Karstaedt A, Venter WD, Omar T, King P, Mbengo T, et al. Causes of death in hospitalized adults with a premortem diagnosis of tuberculosis: an autopsy study. Aids. 2007 Oct 1;21(15):2043-50.

[89] Ikeogu MO, Wolf B, Mathe S. Pulmonary manifestations in HIV seropositivity and malnutrition in Zimbabwe. Arch Dis Child. 1997 Feb;76(2):124-8.

[90] Jeena PM, Coovadia HM, Chrystal V. Pneumocystis carinii and cytomegalovirus infections in severely ill, HIV-infected African infants. Ann Trop Paediatr. 1996 Dec;16(4):361-8.

[91] Beadsworth MB, Cohen D, Ratcliffe L, Jenkins N, Taylor W, Campbell F, et al. Autopsies in HIV: still identifying missed diagnoses. Int J STD AIDS. 2009 Feb;20(2):84-6.

[92] Mudenda V, Lucas S, Shibemba A, O'Grady J, Bates M, Kapata N, et al. Tuberculosis and Tuberculosis/HIV/AIDS-Associated Mortality in Africa: The Urgent Need to Expand and Invest in Routine and Research Autopsies. J Infect Dis. 2012 Mar 23.

[93] WHO. World Health Statistics. 2010.

[94] Gray DM, Zar HJ. Community-acquired pneumonia in HIV-infected children: a global perspective. Curr Opin Pulm Med. 2010 May;16(3):208-16.

[95] Preidis GA, McCollum ED, Mwansambo C, Kazembe PN, Schutze GE, Kline MW. Pneumonia and malnutrition are highly predictive of mortality among African children hospitalized with human immunodeficiency virus infection or exposure in the era of antiretroviral therapy. J Pediatr. Sep; 159(3):484-9.

[96] McNally LM, Jeena PM, Gajee K, Thula SA, Sturm AW, Cassol S, et al. Effect of age, polymicrobial disease, and maternal HIV status on treatment response and cause of severe pneumonia in South African children: a prospective descriptive study. Lancet. 2007 Apr 28;369(9571):1440-51.

[97] Enarson PM, Gie RP, Enarson DA, Mwansambo C, Graham SM. Impact of HIV on standard case management for severe pneumonia in children. Expert Rev Respir Med. 2010 Apr;4(2):211-20.

[98] Nantanda R, Hildenwall H, Peterson S, Kaddu-Mulindwa D, Kalyesubula I, Tumwine JK. Bacterial aetiology and outcome in children with severe pneumonia in Uganda. Ann Trop Paediatr. 2008 Dec;28(4):253-60.

[99] Rabie H, de Boer A, van den Bos S, Cotton MF, Kling S, Goussard P. Children with human immunodeficiency virus infection admitted to a paediatric intensive care unit in South Africa. J Trop Pediatr. 2007 Aug; 53(4):270-3.

[100] Jeena P. The role of HIV infection in acute respiratory infections among children in Sub-Saharan Africa. Int J Tuberc Lung Dis. 2005 Jul;9(7):708-15.

[101] Pillay T, Adhikari M, Mokili J, Moodley D, Connolly C, Doorasamy T, et al. Severe, rapidly progressive human immunodeficiency virus type 1 disease in newborns with coinfections. Pediatr Infect Dis J. 2001 Apr;20(4): 404-10.

[102] Delport SD, Brisley T. Aetiology and outcome of severe community-acquired pneumonia in children admitted to a paediatric intensive care unit. S Afr Med J. 2002 Nov;92(11):907-11.

[103] Punpanich W, Groome M, Muhe L, Qazi SA, Madhi SA. Systematic review on the etiology and antibiotic treatment of pneumonia in human immunodeficiency virus-infected children. Pediatr Infect Dis J. 2011 Oct; 30(10):e192-202.

[104] Ruffini DD, Madhi SA. The high burden of Pneumocystis carinii pneumonia in African HIV-1-infected children hospitalized for severe pneumonia. AIDS. 2002 Jan 4;16(1):105-12.

[105] Graham SM. Impact of HIV on childhood respiratory illness: differences between developing and developed countries. Pediatr Pulmonol. 2003 Dec; 36(6):462-8.

[106] Zampoli M, Morrow B, Hsiao NY, Whitelaw A, Zar HJ. Prevalence and outcome of cytomegalovirus-associated pneumonia in relation to human immunodeficiency virus infection. Pediatr Infect Dis J. 2010 May;30(5):413-7.

[107] Goussard P, Kling S, Gie RP, Nel ED, Heyns L, Rossouw GJ, et al. CMV pneumonia in HIV-infected ventilated infants. Pediatr Pulmonol. 2010 Jul; 45(7):650-5.

[108] Mosca F, Pugni L. Cytomegalovirus infection: the state of the art. J Chemother. 2007 Oct;19 Suppl 2:46-8.

[109] Fowler KB, Stagno S, Pass RF, Britt WJ, Boll TJ, Alford CA. The outcome of congenital cytomegalovirus infection in relation to maternal antibody status. N Engl J Med. 1992 Mar 5;326(10):663-7.

[110] Barbi M, Binda S, Caroppo S, Calvario A, Germinario C, Bozzi A, et al. Multicity Italian study of congenital cytomegalovirus infection. Pediatr Infect Dis J. 2006 Feb;25(2):156-9.

[111] Stagno S, Pass RF, Cloud G, Britt WJ, Henderson RE, Walton PD, et al. Primary cytomegalovirus infection in pregnancy. Incidence, transmission to fetus, and clinical outcome. Jama. 1986 Oct 10;256(14):1904-8.

[112] Griffiths PD, Walter S. Cytomegalovirus. Curr Opin Infect Dis. 2005 Jun; 18(3):241-5.

[113] Kenneson A, Cannon MJ. Review and meta-analysis of the epidemiology of congenital cytomegalovirus (CMV) infection. Rev Med Virol. 2007 Jul-Aug;17(4):253-76.

[114] Gaytant MA, Steegers EA, Semmekrot BA, Merkus HM, Galama JM. Congenital cytomegalovirus infection: review of the epidemiology and outcome. Obstet Gynecol Surv. 2002 Apr;57(4):245-56.

[115] Ross DS, Dollard SC, Victor M, Sumartojo E, Cannon MJ. The epidemiology and prevention of congenital cytomegalovirus infection and disease: activities of the Centers for Disease Control and Prevention Workgroup. J Womens Health (Larchmt). 2006 Apr;15(3):224-9.

[116] Nigro G, Adler SP, La Torre R, Best AM. Passive immunization during pregnancy for congenital cytomegalovirus infection. N Engl J Med. 2005 Sep 29;353(13):1350-62.

[117] Stagno S, Pass RF, Reynolds DW, Moore MA, Nahmias AJ, Alford CA. Comparative study of diagnostic procedures for congenital cytomegalovirus infection. Pediatrics. 1980 Feb;65(2):251-7.

[118] Gibson CS, MacLennan AH, Goldwater PN, Haan EA, Priest K, Dekker GA. Neurotropic viruses and cerebral palsy: population based case-control study. BMJ. 2006 Jan 14;332(7533):76-80.

[119] Schopfer K, Lauber E, Krech U. Congenital cytomegalovirus infection in newborn infants of mothers infected before pregnancy. Arch Dis Child. 1978 Jul;53(7):536-9.

[120] Watts TE, Larsen SA, Brown ST. A case-control study of stillbirths at a teaching hospital in Zambia, 1979-80: serological investigations for selected infectious agents. Bull World Health Organ. 1984;62(5):803-8.

[121] Bos P, Steele D, Alexander J. Prevalence of antibodies to rubella, herpes simplex 2 and cytomegalovirus in pregnant women and in neonates at Ga-Rankuwa. Cent Afr J Med. 1995 Jan;41(1):14-7.

[122] Mostad SB, Kreiss JK, Ryncarz A, Chohan B, Mandaliya K, Ndinya-Achola J, et al. Cervical shedding of herpes simplex virus and cytomegalovirus throughout the menstrual cycle in women infected with human immunodeficiency virus type 1. Am J Obstet Gynecol. 2000 Oct;183(4):948-55.

[123] Mohlala BK, Tucker TJ, Besser MJ, Williamson C, Yeats J, Smit L, et al. Investigation of HIV in amniotic fluid from HIV-infected pregnant women at full term. J Infect Dis. 2005 Aug 1;192(3):488-91.

[124] van der Sande MA, Kaye S, Miles DJ, Waight P, Jeffries DJ, Ojuola OO, et al. Risk factors for and clinical outcome of congenital cytomegalovirus infection in a peri-urban West-African birth cohort. PLoS One. 2007;2(6):e492.

[125] Gerna G, Lilleri D, Furione M, Baldanti F. Management of human cytomegalovirus infection in transplantation: validation of virologic cut-offs for preemptive therapy and immunological cut-offs for protection. New Microbiol. 2011 Jul;34(3):229-54.

[126] Brantsaeter AB, Holberg-Petersen M, Jeansson S, Goplen AK, Bruun JN. CMV quantitative PCR in the diagnosis of CMV disease in patients with HIV-infection - a retrospective autopsy based study. BMC Infect Dis. 2007;7:127.

[127] Erhabor O, Adias TC. From whole blood to component therapy: the economic, supply/demand need for implementation of component therapy in Sub-Saharan Africa. Transfus Clin Biol. 2011 Dec;18(5-6):516-26.

[128] Adler MW. Antiretrovirals for developing world. Lancet. 1998 Jan 24;351(9098):232.

[129] Kober K, Van Damme W. Scaling up access to antiretroviral treatment in southern Africa: who will do the job? Lancet. 2004 Jul 3-9;364(9428):103-7.

[130] Lynch S, Ford N, van Cutsem G, Bygrave H, Janssens B, Decroo T, et al. Public health. Getting HIV treatment to the most people. Science. 2012 Jul 20;337(6092):298-300.

[131] Sharland M, Luck S, Griffiths P, Cotton M. Antiviral therapy of CMV disease in children. Adv Exp Med Biol. 2010;697:243-60.

[132] Mphahlele MJ, Mda S. Immunising the HIV-infected child: A view from Sub-Saharan Africa. Vaccine. 2012 Sep 7;30 Suppl 3:C61-5.

[133] Janaszek W, Gay NJ, Gut W. Measles vaccine efficacy during an epidemic in 1998 in the highly vaccinated population of Poland. Vaccine. 2003 Jan 17;21(5-6):473-8.

[134] Lynn TV, Beller M, Funk EA, Middaugh JP, Ritter D, Rota PA, et al. Incremental effectiveness of 2 doses of measles-containing vaccine compared with 1 dose among high school students during an outbreak. J Infect Dis. 2004 May 1;189 Suppl 1:S86-90.

[135] Vitek CR, Aduddell M, Brinton MJ, Hoffman RE, Redd SC. Increased protections during a measles outbreak of children previously vaccinated with a second dose of measles-mumps-rubella vaccine. Pediatr Infect Dis J. 1999 Jul;18(7):620-3.

[136] Aaby P, Knudsen K, Jensen TG, Tharup J, Poulsen A, Sodemann M, et al. Measles incidence, vaccine efficacy, and mortality in two urban Afri-

can areas with high vaccination coverage. J Infect Dis. 1990 Nov;162(5): 1043-8.

[137] Cisse B, Aaby P, Simondon F, Samb B, Soumare M, Whittle H. Role of schools in the transmission of measles in rural Senegal: implications for measles control in developing countries. Am J Epidemiol. 1999 Feb 15;149(4):295-301.

[138] Malfait P, Jataou IM, Jollet MC, Margot A, De Benoist AC, Moren A. Measles epidemic in the urban community of Niamey: transmission patterns, vaccine efficacy and immunization strategies, Niger, 1990 to 1991. Pediatr Infect Dis J. 1994 Jan;13(1):38-45.

[139] Usen S, Milligan P, Ethevenaux C, Greenwood B, Mulholland K. Effect of fever on the serum antibody response of Gambian children to Haemophilus influenzae type b conjugate vaccine. Pediatr Infect Dis J. 2000 May; 19(5):444-9.

[140] Williamson WA, Greenwood BM. Impairment of the immune response to vaccination after acute malaria. Lancet. 1978 Jun 24;1(8078):1328-9.

[141] Lalor MK, Floyd S, Gorak-Stolinska P, Ben-Smith A, Weir RE, Smith SG, et al. BCG vaccination induces different cytokine profiles following infant BCG vaccination in the UK and Malawi. J Infect Dis. 2011 Oct 1;204(7): 1075-85.

[142] Botha MH, Dochez C. Introducing human papillomavirus vaccines into the health system in South Africa. Vaccine. 2012 Sep 7;30 Suppl 3:C28-34.

[143] Moss WJ, Clements CJ, Halsey NA. Immunization of children at risk of infection with human immunodeficiency virus. Bull World Health Organ. 2003;81(1):61-70.

[144] Simani OE, Leroux-Roels G, Francois G, Burnett RJ, Meheus A, Mphahlele MJ. Reduced detection and levels of protective antibodies to hepatitis B vaccine in under 2-year-old HIV positive South African children at a paediatric outpatient clinic. Vaccine. 2009 Jan 1;27(1):146-51.

[145] Sinzger C, Digel M, Jahn G. Cytomegalovirus cell tropism. Curr Top Microbiol Immunol. 2008;325:63-83.

[146] Sinzger C, Grefte A, Plachter B, Gouw AS, The TH, Jahn G. Fibroblasts, epithelial cells, endothelial cells and smooth muscle cells are major targets of human cytomegalovirus infection in lung and gastrointestinal tissues. J Gen Virol. 1995 Apr;76 (Pt 4):741-50.

[147] Miles DJ, van der Sande M, Jeffries D, Kaye S, Ismaili J, Ojuola O, et al. Cytomegalovirus infection in Gambian infants leads to profound CD8 T-cell differentiation. J Virol. 2007 Jun;81(11):5766-76.

[148] Miles DJ, van der Sande M, Jeffries D, Kaye S, Ojuola O, Sanneh M, et al. Maintenance of large subpopulations of differentiated CD8 T-cells two years after cytomegalovirus infection in Gambian infants. PLoS One. 2008;3(8):e2905.

[149] Trzonkowski P, Mysliwska J, Szmit E, Wieckiewicz J, Lukaszuk K, Brydak LB, et al. Association between cytomegalovirus infection, enhanced proinflammatory response and low level of anti-hemagglutinins during the anti-influenza vaccination--an impact of immunosenescence. Vaccine. 2003 Sep 8;21(25-26):3826-36.

[150] Appay V, Fastenackels S, Katlama C, Ait-Mohand H, Schneider L, Guihot A, et al. Old age and anti-cytomegalovirus immunity are associated with altered T-cell reconstitution in HIV-1-infected patients. AIDS. 2011 Sep 24;25(15):1813-22.

[151] Miles DJ, Sanneh M, Holder B, Crozier S, Nyamweya S, Touray ES, et al. Cytomegalovirus infection induces T-cell differentiation without impairing antigen-specific responses in Gambian infants. Immunology. 2008 Jul; 124(3):388-400.

[152] Holder B, Miles DJ, Kaye S, Crozier S, Mohammed NI, Duah NO, et al. Epstein-Barr virus but not cytomegalovirus is associated with reduced vaccine antibody responses in Gambian infants. PLoS One. 2010;5(11):e14013.

[153] Ben-Smith A, Gorak-Stolinska P, Floyd S, Weir RE, Lalor MK, Mvula H, et al. Differences between naive and memory T cell phenotype in Malawian and UK adolescents: a role for Cytomegalovirus? BMC Infect Dis. 2008;8:139.

[154] Ferlay J SH, Bray F, Forman D, Mathers C,, DM P. Cancer Incidence and Mortality Worldwide. GLOBOCAN 2008 v1.2; 2008 [updated 2008; cited 2012 24th August]; Available from: http://globocan.iarc.fr/.

Chapter 3

Management of CMV-Associated Diseases in Immunocompromised Patients

A.L. Corona-Nakamura and
M.J. Arias-Merino

Additional information is available at the end of the chapter

http://dx.doi.org/10.5772/56141

1. Introduction

Among the great advances that have been achieved in infectious diseases has been on the management of cytomegalovirus (CMV) infection and disease.

This chapter describe an overview of the clinical manifestations of CMV diseases that are in immunocompromised patients, including patients with human immunodeficiency virus infection / Acquired Immunodeficiency Syndrome (HIV / AIDS), organ transplant recipients, bone marrow transplant recipients, and individuals receiving immunosuppressive therapy or chemotherapeutic agents. We also present the conditions for the development of CMV disease in these patients.

In the overall population, the seroprevalence of CMV (IgG) is 30 to 100%. CMV disease is a major cause of death in bone marrow and organ transplant recipients and persons with AIDS. In adult patients with cancer and leukemia (except T cell leukemia) who have not undergone transplantation, the frequency of CMV disease is lower than 3%, but mortality can reach 82% [1-5].

The direct clinical effects of CMV are CMV viral syndrome and end-organ diseases. The indirect effects include superinfections caused by bacteria (eg: *Listeria* or *Pseudomonas*), fungi (eg: *Aspergillus, Pneumocystis jiroveci, Cryptococcus*) or other viruses (herpes zoster, Epstein Barr virus) [6].

2. Terminology

CMV Infection is defined as the detection of the CMV virus by antibodies in blood or the detection of this virus by polymerase chain reaction (PCR), or antigens in any body fluid or tissue specimen, but the infected patient not show any clinical symptoms caused by the virus [2,4,7].

CMV Disease is the presence of CMV infection, evident as:

CMV Syndrome, a clinical condition characterized by fever ≥ 101 ºF (≥ 38.3ºC) at least twice within 7 days, muscle pain, leukopenia ≤ 3500/μl, neutropenia ≤ 1,500/μl, atypical lymphocytosis ≥ 5% and/or thrombocytopenia < 100,000/μl [7] or…

CMV Disease with Organ and Tissue involvement. Clinical presentations [3,4,6] include pneumonitis, gastrointestinal disease (e.g., gastritis, colitis, esophageal ulcers), hepatitis, pancreatitis, nephritis, cystitis, myocarditis, retinitis, central nervous system disease (e.g., meningitis, polyradiculitis, encephalitis, transverse myelitis, Guillain-Barré Syndrome, peripheral neuropathy), thrombocytopenia, hemolytic anemia, adrenalitis, disseminated disease [2].

Primary infection is defined as the detection of CMV infection in an individual previously found to be CMV seronegative. In the case transplanted patients, when the recipient with CMV seronegative (IgG and IgM) receives blood products or a graft from a donor CMV seropositive IgG (D+/R-). The appearance of de novo specific antibodies in a seronegative patient may also be acceptable for the diagnosis of CMV [2,7].

Secondary (Reactivation) infection occurs with the reactivation of endogenous latent CMV, in a CMV seropositive patient, who has (cancer, chronic lymphocytic leukemia, solid organ transplantation, or bone marrow transplantation) with diminished immunity after immunosuppressive therapy or a patient with HIV. The recipient before transplantation is seropositive for CMV (IgG) and the donor is seronegative to CMV (IgG and IgM) (D-/R+) [2,4,8,9]. Reactivation or reinfection again initiates an IgM response. The IgG appears within a few weeks of the IgM rise (4).

Superinfection can occur when the recipient receives a graft or blood products from a donor who is CMV seropositive with different strain of CMV (D+/R+) [2].

Preemptive therapy consists on to monitor weekly by CMV blood PCR to immunocompromised patients and if the test becomes positive, they will be treated with antiviral, irrespective of clinical symptoms. This type of therapy is used in patients with solid organ transplant (specifically with serotypes D+/R +, D-/ R+ and D-/R-), hemopoietic stem cell transplantation, and patient with chronic lymphocytic leukemia who received alemtuzumab, each group of patients has specific guidelines for this type of therapy. Following a study in which CMV DNA was found in 83% of liver transplant recipients at a mean of 13 days before the onset of symptomatic CMV infection, it has become apparent that the preemptive therapy decreases the morbidity and mortality of CMV infection [2].

http://dx.doi.org/10.5772/56141

Prophylactic therapy involves administration of oral valganciclovir or intravenous ganciclovir at-risk patients, such as patients with CMV IgG serostatus negative (D+/R-) or when the recipients need anti-rejection therapy, such as anti-thymocyte globulin (ATG) or anti-lymphocyte globulins (ALGs) [2].

3. The role of immunosuppression

3.1. CMV disease in transplantation recipients

3.1.1. Hemopoietic Stem Cell Transplantation (HSCT)

CMV infections may be more frequently caused by reactivation of the virus in the recipient rather than a primary infection. Approximately 30% of seronegative recipients with seropositive stem cell donors (D+/R-) develop primary CMV infection, whereas reactivation occurs in about 80% who were seropositive before transplantation [8,10].

According the guidelines by Tomblyn *et al* 2009, HSCT recipients at risk for post transplant CMV disease (all CMV-seropositive HSCT recipients, and all CMV-seronegative recipients with a CMV seropositive donor) should have a CMV disease prevention program from the time of transplantation until at least 100 days after HSCT, using prophylaxis or preemptive treatment for allogeneic recipients.

A preemptive strategy against CMV replication (<100 days post-HSCT):

1. To all allogeneic HSCT recipients with evidence of CMV infection for CMV DNA, and this strategy is preferred over prophylaxis therapy for D+/R-. Administer induction doses: Valganciclovir 900 mg twice daily or ganciclovir I.V. 5mg/kg every 12 hours for 7-14 days. Maintenance doses: for another 3-4 weeks until the test is negative or resolution of symptoms.

2. CMV seropositive autologous HSCT recipients with high risk for CMV replication or disease, for example patients who had total body irradiation, and patients who have received alemtuzumab within 6 months prior to HSCT. Administer induction doses: Valganciclovir 900 mg twice daily or ganciclovir I.V. 5mg/kg every 12 hours for 7 days.Maintenance doses: for another 3-4 weeks until the test is negative or resolution of symptoms. Note: Continue screening for CMV reactivation and re-treat if screening tests become positive after discontinuation of therapy [11].

Preemptive therapy > 100 days post-HSCT for:

1. Allogeneic HSCT recipients.

2. All patients receiving steroids for graft-versus-host disease (GVHD), steroid use, low CD4 counts <50/mm^3, and use of grafts from CMV-seronegative donors in CMV-seropositive recipients.

Administer induction doses: Valganciclovir 900 mg twice daily or ganciclovir I.V. 5mg/kg every 12 hours for 7-14 days.

Maintenance doses: for another 3-4 weeks until the test is negative or resolution of symptoms [11].

Prophylactic therapy can be recommended for all allogeneic recipients (from engraftment to 100 days after HSCT), this therapy is not recommended for seropositive autologous recipients, except the patient is at high risk as recipients unrelated, patient with human leucocyte antigen (HLA) system-mismatched or in patients who used the alemtuzumab and are candidates for HSCT. The induction: valganciclovir 450 mg twice daily for 5-7 days. Maintenance: Daily until day 100 after HSCT [8,11,12].

Before the introduction of specific prophylaxis, the risk of CMV disease was reported to be up to 58% in of the allogeneic stem cell transplant seropositive recipients, the clinical presentation more likely was pneumonia with mortality to 94 % [2,7,8,13]. The incidence of CMV pneumonia after autologous bone marrow transplantation and peripheral blood SCT ranges from 1% to 6% [8,14].

Gastrointestinal disease is the most common disease, after CMV pneumonia, which can escape blood-based surveillance by PCR in approximately 25 % of patients. There is presently no consensus on how to use molecular methods to diagnose CMV gastrointestinal and pneumonia disease because there are no data on what level of CMV DNA in brochoalveolar lavage (BAL) fluid or tissue that correlates best with CMV disease. The gastrointestinal disease is treated with antiviral alone. The treatment of CMV pneumonia includes the antiviral and intravenous immunoglobulin. CMV retinitis and encephalitis are rare complications [8,12].

3.1.2. Late CMV disease in HSCT patients

Late CMV disease (after 100 days) occurs in 15% to 20% of seropositive allograft recipients, and it occurs between months 4 and 12 after HSCT, with a mortality rate of 46%. Risk factors for late CMV disease include CMV infection during the first 3 months after transplantation, chronic graft-versus-host disease (GVHD), CD4 counts less 50 per mm3, and undetectable CMV-specific T-cell immunity [8,12].

3.1.3. Solid Organ Transplant (SOT)

CMV infection is most common during the first 3 to 12 weeks after transplantation, this is because in this period is more intense immunosuppression to prevent rejection [2].

There is a high risk of CMV disease when a seronegative receptor receives an organ from a seropositive individual [Donor+/Recipient- (D+/R-)]. Up to 85% of SOT recipients with CMV D+/R- serologic status develop primary CMV disease, with the prophylactic therapy reducing CMV disease to 22% [2].

Other high risk factors are biologic agents used for induction therapy or rejection treatment. These include T lymphocyte (OKT3) monoclonal antibody, ATG, ALGs, or high doses of corticosteroids [2,7].

There is an Intermediate risk of CMV disease with D+/R+ or D-/R+ combinations and a low risk when the donor and recipient are CMV seronegative [2,7].

In kidney transplant patients, 8-18 % will have CMV infection. The clinical presentations may be asymptomatic, fever or affect the transplanted organ, as a glomerulopathy or nephritis [2,7,15].

Amongst liver transplant patients, 29% present CMV infection manifesting as CMV hepatitis [2,6].

Amongst heart transplant patients, 25% present with CMV infection manifesting as myocarditis [2,7]. Of the patients transplanted kidney-pancreas, 50% will present CMV infection usually affecting the transplanted pancreas [2,7].

22% of patients with transplanted small bowel will have CMV infection affecting the transplanted bowel [2,7].

Around 39% of patients with heart-lung transplants can be expected to have CMV infection, usually affecting the lung causing pneumonitis [2,7].

3.1.4. Late CMV disease in solid organ transplanted patients

Antiviral prophylaxis is highly effective in preventing CMV disease in transplanted recipients, particularly in D+/R- patients. However, late-onset CMV disease may occur after 100 days or several years after transplantation, coinciding with discontinuation of antiviral prophylaxis. Among kidney and kidney-pancreas transplant recipients, late-onset CMV disease was documented in 47% of D+/R- patients, 12% of D+/R+ patients, 7% of D-/R+ patients, and 4% of D-/R- patients [16]. One study reported that up to 27% of high-risk (CMV D+/R-) liver and kidney transplantation recipients who received oral ganciclovir prophylaxis for 3 months developed late-onset CMV disease after the completion of antiviral prophylaxis. CMV retinitis and CMV colitis tend to be later manifestations of disease or a clinical presentation atypical [2,16].

In a systematic review, CMV disease occurred in 2.6% and 9.9% of SOT recipients receiving valganciclovir as preemptive therapy and prophylaxis, respectively. In patients receiving valganciclovir prophylaxis, the incidence of early-onset (≤ 90 days posttransplant) CMV disease was 0.8% and 1.2% in all patients (D+/R+, D-/R+) and D+/R- patients, respectively. In the prophylactic group, the incidence of late-onset (>90 days posttransplant) CMV disease rose up to 8.9 % and 17.7 % in all patients and D+/R-, respectively. Ninety-two percent of the patients with CMV disease in the prophylactic group were late-onset disease. No patients developed late-onset CMV disease in preemptive group. Late-onset CMV disease is a complication observed uniquely with valganciclovir prophylaxis, particularly in D+/R- patients, but not with preemptive therapy [17].

The rejection rate was 10.8% in SOT recipients who receiving preemptive therapy. The overall rejection was 17.6% in the prophylactic studies. Fifteen patients (3.9%) of 380 patients in preemptive group had graft loss. In prophylactic studies the graft loss rate was 2.5%. The patients who receiving preemptive therapy, 28.5% developed opportunistic infections. In contrast, prophylactic studies reported the proportion of patients with opportunistic infections was 7.8%. The mortality was 8.2% from four preemptive studies, and 4.4% in prophylactic studies [17].

3.1.5. Recurrent CMV disease

Recurrent CMV disease may occur in up to 25% of SOTR (2). Predictive factors include the type of organ transplant, CMV DNA in plasma at day 21, negative CMV IgG serostatus D+/R- at start of treatment and therapy for acute rejection (18). The rate of recurrent CMV disease for lung transplant recipients was 38.5%, for kidney 14.6%, for heart 11.8%, and for liver transplant recipients was 0%. The yearly risk of recurrent CMV disease was 24.4% for patients with persistent CMV DNAemia in plasma at day 21 versus 8.8% for those eradicated at day 21 [18].

CMV recurrence may be related to incomplete suppression of viral replication or the duration of treatment (often 2-4 weeks) may have been insufficient. Some authors suggest treatment for 3 months for pneumonitis, retinitis and gastrointestinal CMV disease. Plasma levels of CMV DNA should influence the therapy duration [2]. Weekly monitoring until eradication is recommended [18].

3.2. CMV disease in patients with HIV/AIDS

CMV infection was one of the most important opportunistic infection in HIV-infected patients before the introduction of the highly active antiretroviral therapy. Approximately 40% of HIV-infected patients with advanced disease suffered from one of several manifestations of CMV infection during their life. Colitis is the second most common presentation of CMV disease after CMV retinitis (4). It is related to the degree of T-cell impairment, being most common in patients with $CD4^+$ T-cell counts bellow 50-100 cells/μl [3,19].

3.3. CMV disease in patients with rheumatic diseases

The incidence of CMV in rheumatic patients was 50% for systemic lupus erythematosus (SLE), 10% for dermatomyositis, 8.8% for microscopic polyangitis, and less than 5% for rheumatoid arthritis, rheumatoid vasculitis, Behcet´s disease, Chung-Strauss syndrome. The mortality rates CMV disease were 20-75% rheumatological disease depending on the type. The fever was the most common symptom, respiratory symptoms were the second most common, followed by gastrointestinal symptoms. Visual disturbance was observed in one patient [20].

CMV infection was most common among patients under strong immunosupressive therapy (eg: 500-1000 mg pulsed methylprednisolone per day, 60-100 mg oral prednisolone, or intravenous or oral cyclophosphamide within a year before CMV diagnosis [19]. The effect of corticosteroid involves derangement of T lymphocyte and monocyte/macrophage functions, and blockade of the production of cytokines such as TNF-α. Cyclophosphamide suppresses lymphocyte proliferation and function which increasing the risk of CMV reactivation and replication [1,20-22].

3.4. CMV disease in patients with haematological malignancies and solid tumours

CMV disease is potentiated by drugs that cause profound cell-mediated immunosuppression, such as fludarabine (which depresses CD4 T-lymphocytes), high-dose cyclophosphamide, high-dose of steroids and granulocyte transfusions from donors who have CMV disease, and with the use of metotrexate, cyclosporine, alemtuzumab (anti-CD52 MoAb) and rituximab (anti-CD20 MoAb). The mortality rate among the patients with leukemia, myelodysplastic syndrome or lymphoma was 82%, and the 63% of the fatal cases was due to, relapse of leukemia, refractory leukemia, or that these patients were in accelerated or blast phase [1,23].

In 2001, serious CMV disease, (primarily pneumonia) was found at autopsy in 17%-75% of patients dying with T cell leukemia. Mortality was higher among patients who had lymphopenia [1].

3.4.1. Guidelines on the management of CMV reactivation in patients with chronic lymphocytic leukemia treated with alemtuzumab

Chronic lymphocytic leukemia (CLL) is a disease of progressive with an accumulation of clonal B lymphocytes in peripheral blood, marrow, and lymphoid organs. This is generally incurable, except the patients who receive an allogeneic cell transplant, and it is the most common form of adult leukemia in Western countries. Patients with CLL have impaired humoral and cellular immunity [24-26]. Current treatments for patients with CLL include monoclonal antibodies (eg. rituximab and alemtuzumab) among others [9,27].

Alentuzumab is a recombinant humanized, anti-CD52 monoclonal antibody with significant activity in CLL, including frudarabine-refractory disease. CD52 is a glycoprotein of unknown function that is expressed on the surfaces of normal and malignant B and T lymphocytes. Binding of alemtuzumab to CD52 on lymphocytes induces complement-dependent cytotoxicity, antibody-dependent cell-mediated cytotoxicity (which results in a rapid and profound reduction of lymphocytes, and this produces viral replication and reactivation CMV) and direct cytotoxicity (likely apoptotic cell death) [9,24,25,27-29].

Viral infections often are presented at the third week after the initiation of alemtuzumab, which coincides with the nadir in T-cell numbers. The CMV reactivation is the most common opportunistic infection observed in alemtuzumab-treated patients and it is observed at the beginning of the 4 - 6 weeks of alemtuzumab [30]. O´Brien *et al* estimated the incidence of CMV reactivation ranges from 4 to 30 %. This incidence typically refers to symptomatic CMV infection [9,24,28,31,32]. CMV pneumonitis was reported 0.8 %, and CMV-related death 0.2 %. CMV reactivation which frequently presents as fever of unknown origin or respiratory symptoms [9,24,28,31,33].

Updated management guidelines for using alemtuzumab in CLL.

Among the recommendations on the use of alemtuzumab in the patient with CLL, is monitoring for opportunistic infections, such as CMV reactivation, theses management guidelines are referred by Osterborg A *et al*, 2009, and O'Brien *et al* 2006 for monitoring and treating of CMV reactivation, such as:

1. Baseline CMV serology prior to therapy of the patient
2. If the fever unresponsive to antibacterial agents and test not available should be presumed to be CMV reactivation and the alemtuzumab should discontinue and antiviral therapy should start [9,24,25,27,28,31]
3. Monitoring CMV reactivation by weekly PCR during therapy, and every 2 weeks for 6 weeks after alemtuzumab discontinuation [34-36].

If the CMV PCR two consecutive positive results obtained 1 week apart, it should start preemptive therapy with intravenous ganciclovir or oral valganciclovir or when CMV reactivation becomes symptomatic or viremia increase, alemtuzumab therapy should be interrupted and anti-CMV therapy to be started (Figure 1) [9,24,25,28].

The antiviral is administrated 900 mg twice daily for 21 days, or continue with the maintenance dose 900 mg twice daily until the CMV PCR is negative or until you have 2 consecutive negative results [9,24,25,28].

The pre-emptive treatment prevents the occurrence of potentially life-threatening infectious diseases, and the initiation of anti-CMV treatment avoids the interruption of alemtuzumab [31].

Another modality is the anti-CMV prophylaxis in CLL patients receiving alemtuzumab, is with valganciclovir 450 mg twice daily. The prophylaxis is administrated entire duration of Alemtuzumab therapy and until 2 months after end the therapy and the frequency of CMV PCR is every 2 weeks. The valganciclovir prophylaxis may be used in patients with elevated risk for CMV reactivation [9, 28]. Patients on prophylactic valganciclovir had a lower rate of CMV activation compared with valacyclovir (3% vs 24%) among patients being treated with an alemtuzumab-based regimen [26,32]

3.5. CMV infection in patients with inflammatory bowel disease

CMV disease is seen in patients under treatment with azathioprine alone or with 5-aminosalicylic acid, steroids, and/or infliximab, or 6-mercaptopurine, or leukocytapheresis. Crohn disease (CD) was underlying disease in 77% of cases possibly because immunosuppression is more common in CD compared to Ulcerative colitis (UC) [6].

4. Clinical presentations of CMV disease

4.1. CMV Pneumonia (CMVp)

"CMVp" is defined as the occurrence of clinical and radiographic evidence of pneumonia, in association with the isolation of CMV in BAL, or lung-tissue specimens or with the identification of CMV in lung tissue by histopathology, immunohistochemistry or PCR [1].

CMVp represents a major cause of morbidity and mortality in highly immunosuppressed patients, the clinical presentation resembles *Pneumocystis jiroveci* pneumonia (PCP), the

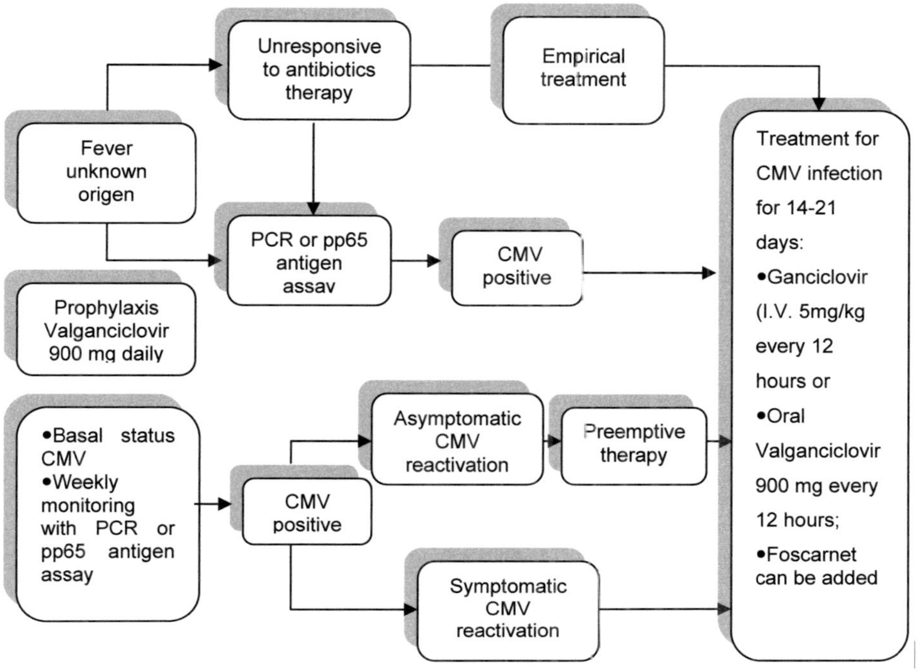

PCR, polymerase chain reaction; IV, via intravenous.

Figure 1. Guidelines on the Management in Cytomegalovirus Monitoring for Patients with Chronic Lymphocytic Leukemia Treated with Alemtuzumab

presence of extrapulmonary CMV disease could suggest the diagnosis of CMV pneumonia [37]. The symptoms are fever, nonproductive cough, dyspnea, or worsening dyspnea that progresses to hypoxemia, and necessitates assisted mechanical ventilation [6]. It can include extrapulmonary CMV disease (gastrointestinal or retinitis) [37]. The signs can include normal breath sounds at auscultation or basal crepitations [6].

On chest radiograph the infiltrates are usually bilateral and may be interstitial and diffuse (figure 2), or nodular, or alveolar and occasionally small pleural effusions [37]. The most common manifestations of CMVp on conventional radiographs are parenchymal consolidation and multiple nodules measuring less 5 mm in diameter [38].

In patients having AIDS, the most frequent finding was dense consolidation and mass-like opacities. The most frequent computed tomography (CT) pattern in immunocompromised patients without AIDS was ground-glass opacities which were bilateral patchy, diffuse distribution. Other findings included poorly-defined small nodules and consolidation. Interlobular septal thickening and pleural effusion [38,39].

Coinfections were other potentially life-threatening infections that occurred within 90 days of the episode of CMVp. These can contribute to death in patients with fatal CMVp [23].

HSCT and lung transplant recipients who develop CMVp or infection have an increased risk for subsequent invasive aspergillosis [23].

In allogeneic bone marrow transplant recipients, the incidence of CMVp is 20-35% and the mortality is up to 50% [40]. IV ganciclovir is given concurrently with immune serum globulin or hyperimmune globulin. In autologous bone marrow transplant recipients, the incidence of CMVp is 2% [9,23]. The mortality rate from CMVp in patients with HSCT was 100% [23].

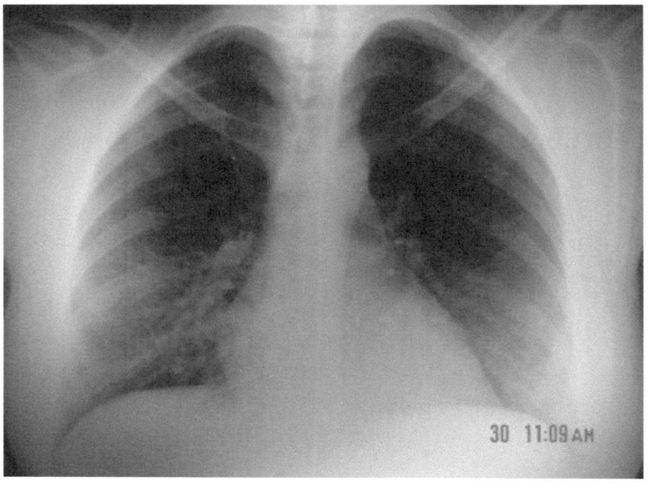

Figure 2. Bilateral interstitial pneumonia caused by CMV in a renal transplant recipient

In solid organ transplantation, the incidence of CMVp is 17 to 90 % [23].

In adults with leukemia, the frequency of CMVp was 0.4%, 2.2%, 2.3%, and 2.5% in patients with myelodysplastic syndrome, acute myelogenous leukemia (AML), chronic myelogenous leukemia (CML), and acute lymphocytic leukemia (ALL) respectively and 8.8% and 11% in patients with chronic lymphocytic leukemia (CLL) and lymphoblastic lymphoma. The median duration of time from the diagnosis of leukemia to the occurrence of CMVp ranged from 6 months and 9 months in patients with AML and ALL, respectively, to 25 months and 54 months in patients with CML, and CLL respectively [1,23].

The CMVp among patients with leukemia, lymphoma and myelodysplastic syndrome, the mortality rate was 57%, and the death occurred 15 (2-36) days after onset of illness. Among patients treated before the occurrence of respiratory failure, the mortality rate was 48%. When therapy was initiated after the occurrence of respiratory failure that required mechanical ventilation, the mortality rate was 57-100 % [1,23].

Chemaly *et al.* [23] observed that, the incidence of CMVp among adults with lymphoma was 0.6-1.2%. In the 92% of the patients, chemotherapy had been administered to the patients within 6 months before the onset of CMVp. Essentially, these patients with lymphoma were treated with rituximab or alemtuzumab [23].

A study of cancer patients receiving chemotherapy placed the incidence of CMVp below 3%, in patients with head and neck cancers, nasopharyngeal cancer (NPC), hypopharyngeal cancer (HPC), lung cancer, lymphoma and rectal cancer. The chemotherapy regimen used was cisplatin, 5-FU, fluorouracil, leucovorin and etoposide. As the incidence is low, prophylactic therapy was not recommended [5].

Cascio *et al.* [6] reported that the 85% of patients with inflammatory bowel disease who developed CMVp were on treatment with thiopurines (azathioprine and 6-mercaptopurine) when they developed CMVp. The mean length of treatment with azathioprine before the appearance of respiratory symptoms was 19 months, with 6-mercaptopurine was 18 months, infliximab was 10 days to 3 weeks, and cyclosporine was 3 days. These patients had hematological findings such as pancytopenia, lymphopenia, neutropenia, leucopenia, severe anemia, hemophagocytic lymphohistiocytosis or thrombocytopenia. Symptoms lasted from 2 days to 1 month [6,23].

4.2. CMV gastrointestinal (GI) diseases

Symptoms range from low-grade fever, weight loss, anorexia, abdominal pain, and bloody diarrhea to a fulminant colitis. In HIV patients can have present esophageal ulcer, esophagitis, gastritis, duodenitis, jejunal and ileal perforation, peritonitis secondary, odynophagia, and bowel obstruction. GI CMV disease is estimated to affect about 20% of adults with AIDS, and it can be involved all parts of the gastrointestinal tract, but the colon and esophagus are the most common sites [4, 41]. CMV infection of the endothelial cells and ensuing vasculitis may play a role in the development of thrombosis, local ischemia and ulceration of the gastrointestinal mucosa [41].

4.2.1. CMV colitis

Refers to the presence of the virus in the colon in sites of inflamed tissue. Within patients with severe ulcerative colitis (UC), CMV disease may occur more commonly in patients over age 55, and in patients treated with steroids. Steroids produce suppression of CMV-specific T-cell function. Infliximab has not been associated with an increased risk of CMV in patients with inflammatory bowel disease (IBD) [4].

The prevalence of CMV colitis in resected IBD specimens ranged from 0 to 22% [39], the prevalence assessed using CMV DNA in colon biopsy was 81% in UC patients, and 66% prevalence in Crohn ′s disease patients [3]. Domenech *et al*, showed a prevalence of colonic CMV of 32% in patients with steroid-refractory UC [10].

CMV colitis has occurred primarily in patients with pre-existing UC, with documented disease for as long as 20-30 years [3]. Another theory was that CMV was an innocent bystander in IBD colitis. This may reflect infection with nonpathogenic genotypes. The challenge is differentiating the innocent bystanders from the pathogenic strains, so most patients are treated with antivirals, as the possible cost of delaying antiviral therapy is colectomy or even death. Refractory IBD colitis have been associated with CMV inclusions bodies, and these patients have a colectomy rate of 62% and a mortality rate of 44% [3].

CMV reactivation exacerbates disease severity in those with active intestinal inflammation. Patients with IBD have impaired NK cell activity and defects in mucosal immunity, which may enhance susceptibility to CMV reactivation). Patients described as "steroid-refractory" show CMV detectable by immunohistochemistry (IHC) in 20%-40% of both endoscopic biopsies and colectomy specimens. CMV DNA was detectable in the colon of up to 60% of patients in the same study [4].

CMV colitis is rare in patients with Crohn´s disease or mild-moderate ulcerative colitis. In patients with severe and/or steroid-refractory ulcerative colitis, the possibility of a concurrent CMV infection causing or worsening the colitis is considered, especially when patients are on immunosuppressive medications. Local reactivation of CMV can be detected in actively inflamed colonic tissue in about 30% of cases [3].

CMV has tropism for dysplastic colonic tissue (adenomas and adenocarcinomas) and may play a significant role in cancer progression. The association of CMV infection with dysplasia progression in IBD patients increases the risk of developing colorectal cancer [3].

The diagnosis includes:

Endoscopic findings comprise patchy erythema, exudates, microerosions, edematous mucosa, or deep ulcers and pseudotumor [42]. These findings can be very difficult to distinguish from severe IBD colitis [39]. CMV colitis may exclusively affect the right colon in up to 30% of cases [3].

CMV antigenemia is being supplanted by leukocyte CMV PCR. A "cut off" level of viremia for distinguishing infection from disease is required for CMV colitis in patients with IBD [4]. Higher CMV viral loads correlate with symptomatic disease [3]. Most studies in patients with IBD have reported a correlation between identification of CMV by PCR in blood, and colonic detection in tissue by hematoxylin and eosin (H&E) or IHC [3,4]. IHC improves histological sensitivity. It uses monoclonal antibodies, identifying infected cells in the colon. Sensibility ranges 78%-93% [4]. PCR of colonic tissue can be used to detect viral DNA [5]. The GI disease can occur even if there is no detection of CMV in the blood [10].

The European Crohn´s and Colitis Organization guidelines (2009) [4]: its authors recommend the use of tissue PCR or IHC in investigating for CMV in cases of IBD.

Guidelines from the American College of Gastroenterology, and the European Crohn´s & Colitis Organization (ECCO) recommend treatment with antivirals when CMV is detected by blood PCR or IHC on colonic biopsies, which must be performed in all patients with severe colitis refractory to immunosuppressive therapy. They do not recommend colonic PCR because they give false positive results. Likewise, they recommend the discontinuation of immunosuppressive agents only in cases of severe systemic CMV disease[4].

Treatment with antiviral therapy has allowed some patients with severe colitis to avoid colectomy despite poor response to conventional IBD therapies. CMV colitis is usually treated with ganciclovir, foscarnet, valganciclovir, or cidofovir. The recommended dosage is for at least 3-6 weeks. The "response rate" in patients with steroid-refractory disease who have reactivation of CMV is 72% (range 50%-100%) (figure 3) [3, 4].

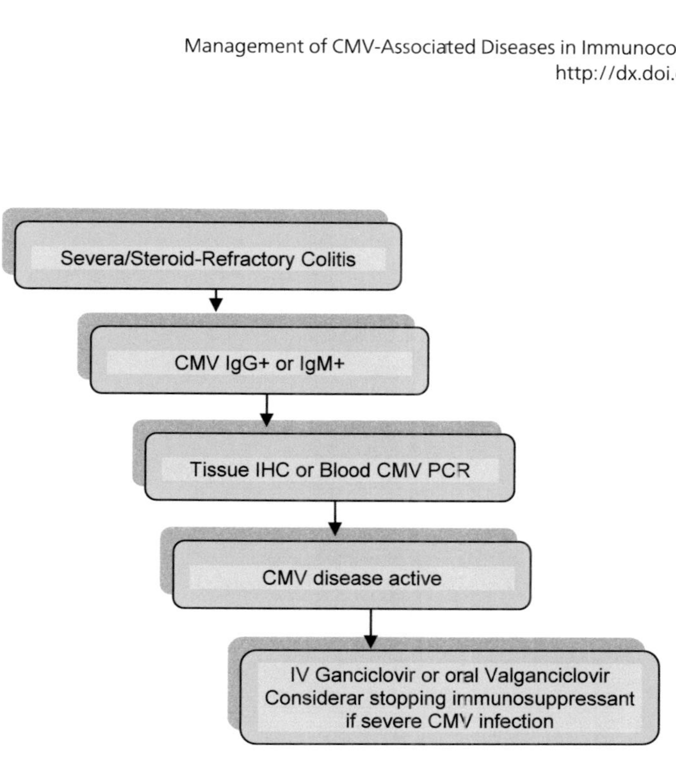

Figure 3. Algorithm for management of suspected CMV colitis in patients with IBD [4]

In patients having AIDS, relapse of CMV gastrointestinal disease in AIDS patients can occur between 9 week and 1 year after initial antiviral [3].

4.2.2. CMV hepatitis

Is defined by findings such as fever, vomiting, with hepatomegaly with hepatalgia, and atypical lymphocytosis may be approximately 50%, elevated bilirubin and/or enzyme levels, and detection of CMV by histopathologic analysis within the liver tissue is needed [13,42].

4.2.3. CMV pancreatitis

Requires the detection of CMV infection by immunohistochemical analysis together with the identification in a pancreatic biopsy. Detection of CMV by PCR alone is insufficient for diagnosis of CMV pancreatitis because it can imply the presence of transient viremia [42].

4.3. CMV retinitis

Retinitis can appear more than 6 months after solid organ transplantation, mainly heart transplant recipients. The patients can be asymptomatic, or they may experience blurring of vision, scotomata, or decreased visual acuity. Fundoscopy often reveals the diagnosis [2]. In HIV-infected patients, retinitis is the single most common manifestation of CMV disease, accounting for 85% of all cases. In developing countries, CMV retinitis is still the most frequent cause of visual loss in HIV-infected patients. Accordingly, the incidence of CMV retinitis, which is the most common CMV disease among HIV patients, decreased from 17.1/100 patient years to 5.6/100 patient-years [2, 43].

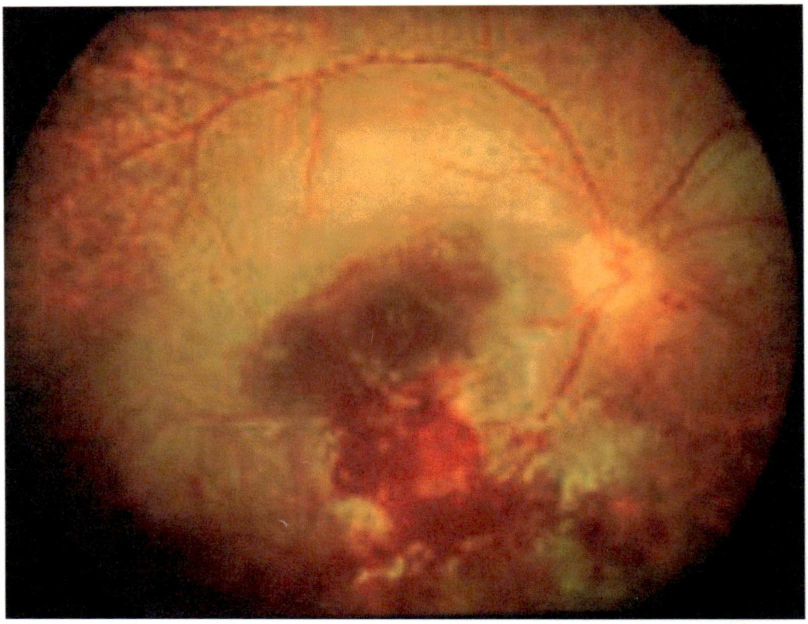

Figure 4. Reference [43]

CMV retinitis in a patient with AIDS appears as an arcuate zone of retinitis with extensive haemorrhages and optic disk swelling (figure 4) [43].

4.4. CMV neurological diseases

4.4.1. CMV Guillain–Barré Syndrome (GBS)

GBS has become the most frequent cause of acute flaccid paralysis in Western countries, following the near-elimination of poliomyelitis. The current annual incidence is estimated to be 0.75–2 cases/100 000 population. Infectious agents have been suggested as possible triggers of GBS, as some form of respiratory or gastrointestinal infection precedes nearly two-thirds of GBS cases. Infection with CMV is the most common antecedent virus infection, as identified by the presence of IgM antibodies in 10–15% of patients at the onset of GBS. However, antiviral therapy is currently not recommended in cases of GBS, since the disease is considered to be post infectious. Recently, the presence of CMV DNA has been demonstrated in almost one-third of serum and cerebrospinal fluid samples from GBS patients who were positive for CMV-specific antibodies at the onset of the neurological disease [43]

http://dx.doi.org/10.5772/56141

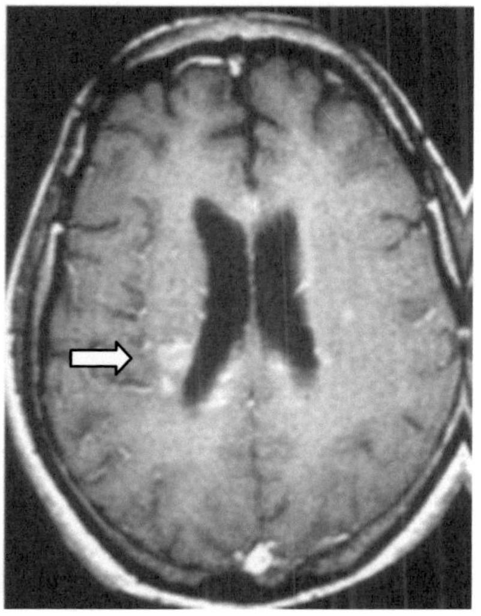

Figure 5. Reference [43]

4.4.2. CMV ventriculoencephalitis

This occurs rarely. It presents with changes in mental function. Multiple small, peri-ventricular lesions of the brain are detected following brain magnetic resonance imaging (arrow) (figure 5) [2,43].

4.5. CMV genitourinary diseases

4.5.1. CMV Nephritis

It can be defined by the detection of CMV infection by immunohistochemical analysis together with the identification of histological features of CMV infection in a kidney biopsy. Detection of CMV by PCR alone is insufficient for this diagnosis [42].

4.5.2. CMV Cystitis

This CMV disease is defined by detection of CMV by immunohistochemical together with identification of conventional histological features of CMV in a bladder biopsy obtained from patient with symptoms of cystitis [42].

4.6. CMV myocarditis

This occurs most frequently in heart transplant recipients. This infection is defined by the detection of CMV infection by immunohistochemical analysis together with the identification of conventional histological features of CMV infection in a heart biopsy specimen and CMV

PCR. Detection of CMV by PCR alone is insufficient for the diagnosis of CMV myocarditis [42]. There is an association between CMV and left ventricular dysfunction [2].

4.7. CMV vasculopathy

The CMV vasculopathy is considered to be an inflammatory disease. CMV and others organisms such as *Chlamydia pneumoniae*, Epstein Barr virus, herpes simplex virus-1, *Mycoplasma pneumoniae* and *Helicobacter pylori* are implicated, but evidence is strongest with CMV and *Chlamydia pneumoniae*. There is a correlation between CMV seropositivity and the presence of atherosclerosis, restenosis following and coronary angioplasty and transplant vascular sclerosis. CMV antigens and nucleic acids have been detected in atherosclerotic lesions in the different layers of the human aorta. Patients suffering from acute myocardial infarction have been found to develop CMV antigenaemia, reflecting either a primary infection or reactivation of a latent infection [44].

CMV infects cells in vessels on endotelial cells, smooth muscle cells and macrophages contribute to the slow progression and aggravation of atherosclerosis. The virus may also contribute to coronary thrombosis [44].

4.8. CMV associated Hemophagocytic Syndrome (HPS)

CMV hemophagocytic syndrome, also referred as macrophage activation syndrome (MAS) or haemophagocytic lymphohistiocytosis (HLH), is a reactive disorder, characterized by generalized histiocytic proliferation, with marked hemophagocytosis. This syndrome was first described by Risdull et al in 1979 in transplant patients [45]. There are two forms of HPS, familial erytrocytic lymphohistiocytosis and the secondary or reactive HPS [34,46,47].

Reactive or secondary HPS may develop during systemic infections, immunodeficiencies or malignancies. Infection-associated hemophagocytic syndrome (IAHS) is observed with viral infections (CMV, Epstein Barr virus, human herpes virus 8, human herpes virus 6, Parvovirus B19 or BK polyoma virus), bacterial infections (*Escherichia coli* and *Mycobacterium*), fungal infection (*Histoplasma, Pneumocystis*, and *Penicillum marneffei*), parasitic infections (toxoplasmosis, leishmaniasis or babesiosis). HPS may also develop as a complication of malignancies such as T-cell lymphomas and metastatic carcinomas. Secundary HPS to inflammatory/ autoimmune disorders, including systemic lupus erythematosus, rheumatoid arthritis and Still´s disease, or due anticonvulsants such as phenytoin and carbamazepine [34,45,46].

Cytomegalovirus has been associated with haemophagocytic syndrome in healthy patients, patients with inflammatory bowel diseases, rheumatological diseases, and transplant recipients [45,47].

The pathophysiology of HPS is not completely understood there is an activation of lymphohistiocytic tissue secondary to hypercytokinemia derived from the activation of T lymphocytes and activated macrophages, causing fever, shock, and organ dysfunction [48,4]).

The HLH (Henter, 2004), (Emmenegger, 2005) diagnostic criteria are shown in Table 1,

http://dx.doi.org/10.5772/56141

The most typical signs of HPS are fever ≥ 38.3ºC) and splenomegaly associated with pancytopenia (affecting ≥ 2 cell lineages in peripheral blood), hepatic enzyme abnormalities, hypertriglyceridemia or hypofibrinogenemia are common features of HPS. The diagnostic sensitivity of hypertriglyceridemia, hypofibrinogenemia and splenomegaly may be about 50%, but the diagnostic sensitivity of low NK cell activity and soluble CD25 levels approaches 100%. The histopathologic features are not pathognomonic. The most prominent feature is proliferation of histiocytes and hemophagocytosis in bone marrow, spleen, or lymph nodes, with no evidence of malignancy [34,45,48,49].

1. Fever: ≥ 101 ºF (≥ 38.3ºC) for more than a week
2. Splenomegaly: about 3 cm below the costal arch
3. Absence of malignancy
4. Cytopenia of ≥ 2 cell lines
Hemoglobin ≤ 9 g/dl, or platelets count < 100,000/µl, or neutrophil count < 1,000/µl
5. Hypertriglyceridemia: Fasting triglycerides ≥ 265 mg/dl (> 3 mmol/l)
6. Hypofibrinogenemia: < 1.5 g/l
7. Serum ferritin > 500 µg/l
8. Hemophagocytosis demonstrated in bone marrow, spleen, or lymph node
9. Low or absent NK cell activity) ≥ 2,400 U/ml
10. Soluble CD25 (soluble interleukin-2 receptor) ≥ 2,400 U/ml

Table 1. HLH-2004 Diagnostic criteria, References [48,49]

Therapy includes corticosteroids, cyclosporine, withdrawal of the immunosuppressant treatment, intravenous immunoglobulins (0.4g/ kg /day for 5 days) and antiviral treatment. The mortality rates are 30-40 % [45]. The hemophagocytic syndrome should be considered if a patient has fever of unknown origin, pancytopenia and multiorgan dysfunction [45,48,49].

Author details

A.L. Corona-Nakamura and M.J. Arias-Merino

From the Infectious Disease Department Specialities Hospital, West Medical Center, Instituto Mexicano del Seguro Social, Guadalajara, Jalisco, México

References

[1] Nguyen Q, Estey E, Radd I, Rolston K, Kantarjian H, Jacobson K, et al. Cytomegalovirus Pneumonia in Adults with Leukemia: An Emerging Problem. *CID* 2001; 32: 539-45.

[2] Paya CV, Razonable RR. Cytomegalovirus Infection after Solid Organ Transplantation. In:Bowden RA, Ljungman P, Paya CV, eds. *Transplant Infections*. 2nd ed. Philadelphia: Lippincott-Raven Publishers; 2003.p. 298-325.

[3] Kandiel A, Lashner B. Cytomegalovirus Colitis Complicating Inflammatory Bowel Disease. *Am J Gastroenterol* 2006; 101: 2857-2865.

[4] Lawlor G, and Moss AC. Clinical Review. Cytomegalovirus in Inflammatory Bowel Disease: Pathogen or Innocent Bystander? *Inflamm Bowel Dis* 2010; 16: 1620-1627.

[5] Kuo CP, Wu CL, Ho HT, Chen CG, Liu SI and Lu YT. Detection of cytomegalovirus reactivation in cáncer patients receiving chemotherapy. *Clin Microbiol Infect* 2008; 14:221-227.

[6] Cascio A, Laria C, Ruggeri P, Fries W. Cytomegalovirus pneumonia in patients with inflammatory bowel disease: a systematic review. *Int J Infect Dis* 16 (2012) e474-e479.

[7] Cytomegalovirus Prophylaxis following Solid Organ Transplants Guideline Team, Cincinnati Children's Hospital Medical Center: Evidence-based care guideline for CMV Prophylaxis following Solid Organ Transplant. Guideline 17, pages 1-16, July 6, 2007. www.cincinnatichildrens.org/svc/alpha/health-policy/ev-based/CMV-Transplant.htm.

[8] Boeckh MJ, Ljungman P. Cytomegalovirus Infection after Hemopoietic Stem Cell Transplantation. In: Bowden RA, Ljungman P, Paya CV, eds. *Transplant Infections*. 2nd ed. Philadelphia: Lippincott-Raven Publishers; 2003.p. 277-397.

[9] O'Brien SM, Keating MJ, Mocarski ES. Updated Guidelines on the Management of Cytomegalovirus Reactivation in Patients with Chronic Lymphocytic Leukemia Treated with Alemtuzumab. *Clin Lymphoma Myelom* 2006; 7 (2): 125-130.

[10] Domenech E, Vega R, Ojanguren I, *et a*l. Cytomegalovirus in Inflammatory Bowel Disease: Time for another look? *Gastroenterology* 2009; 137:1163-1175.

[11] Tomblyn M., Chiller T, Einsele H, Gress R, Sepkowitz K, Storek J, *et al*. Guidelines for Preventing Infectious Complications among Hematopoietic Cell Transplantation Recipients: A Global Perspective. *Biol Blood Marrow Tr* 2009; 15:1143-1148.

[12] Boeckh M. Complications, Diagnosis, Management, and Prevention of CMV Infections: Current and Future. *Hematology* 2011; 305-309.

[13] Crumpacker C. S, Zhang JL. Citomegalovirus. In: Mandell GL, Bennett JE, Dolin R, eds. *Enfermedades Infecciosas. Principios y Práctica*. 7ma. Ed. Barcelona, España: Elsevier; 2012.p.1983-2000.

[14] Kim EA, Lee KS, Primack SL, Yoon HK, Byun HS, Kim TS, *et al*. Viral Pneumonias in Adults: Radiologic and Pathologic Findings. *Radiographics* 2002; 22: S137-S149.

[15] Corona Nakamura AL, Monteón Ramos FJ, Troyo Sanroman R, Arias Merino MJ, Anaya Prado R. Incidence and predictive factors for cytomegalovirus infection in renal transplant recipients. *Transplant Proc* 2009; 41:2412–5.

[16] Kotton CN, and Fishman JA. Disease of the month. Viral Infection in the Renal Transplant Recipient. *J Am Soc Nephrol* 2005; 16, 1758-1774.

[17] Sun H-Y, Wagener MM and Singh N. Prevention of Posttransplant Cytomegalovirus Disease and Related Outcomes with Valganciclovir: A Systematic Review. *Am J Transplant* 2008, 8: 2111-2118.

[18] Asberg A, Humar A, Jardine AG, Rollag H, Pescovitz MD, Mouas H, *et al.* Long-Term Outcomes of CMV Disease Treatment with Valganciclovir Versus IV Ganciclovir in Solid Organ Transplant Recipients. *Am J Transplant* 2009; 9: 1205-1213.

[19] Tamm M. The Lung in the Immunocompromised Patient. Thematic Review Series. *Respiration* 1999; 66: 199-207.

[20] Takizawa Y, Inokuma S, Tanaka Y, Saito K, Atsumi T, Hirakata M, *et al*. Clinical characteristics of cytomegalovirus infection in rheumatic diseases: multicentre survey in a large patient population. *Rheumatology* 2008; 47:1373-1378.

[21] Aries PM, Ullrich S, Gross WL. A case of destructive Wegener´s granulomatosis complicated by cytomegalovirtus infection. *Nature Clinical Practice Rheumatology* 2006; 2: 511-515.

[22] Wade JC. Viral Infection in Patients with Hematological Malignancies. *Am Soc Hematol* 2006; 368-373.

[23] Chemaly RF, Torres HA, Hachem RY, Nogueras GM, Aguilera EA, Younes A, *et al.* Cytomegalovirus Pneumonia in Patients with Lymphoma. Cancer 2005; 104 (6): 1213-1220.

[24] Desai S, PharmD, and Pinilla-Ibarz J. Front-Line Therapy for Chronic Lymphocytic Leukemia. *Cancer Control* 2012; 19 (1): 26-36.

[25] Thursky KA, Worth LJ, Seymour JF, Prince HM, and Slavin MA. Spectrum of infection, risk and recmmendations for prophylaxis and screening among patients with lymphoproliferative disorders treated with alemtuzumab. *Brit J Haematol* 2005; 132: 3-12.

[26] Badoux XC, Keating MJ, Wang X, O'Brien SM, Ferrajoli A, Fadert S, *et al.* Cyclophosphamide, fludarabine, alemtuzuman, and rituximab as salvage therapy for heavily pretreated patients with chronic lymphocytic leukemia. *Blood* 2011; 118 (8): 2085-2092.

[27] Elter T, Hallek M, and Montillo M. Alemtuzumab: What Is the Secret to Safe Therapy?. *Clin Advan Hematol Oncol* 2011; 9 (5): 364-372.

[28] Österborg A, Foá R, Bezares RF, Dearden C. Dyer MJS, Geisler C, Lin TS, *et al.* Review. Management guidelines for the use of alemtuzumab in chronic lymphocytic leukemia. *Leukemia* 2009; 23:1980-1988.

[29] Cortelezzi A, Gritti G, Laurenti L, Cuneo A., Ciolli S, Di Renzo N, *et al.* An Italian retrospective study on the routine clinical use of low-dose alemtuzumab in relapsed/refractory chronic lymphocytic leukemia patients. *Brit J Haematol* 2011; 156:481-489.

[30] Petersen CC, Nederby L, Roug AS, Skovbo A, Peterslund NA, Hokland P, *et al.* Increased Expression of CD69 on T Cells as an Early Immune Marker for Human Cytomegalovirus Reactivation in Chronic Lymphocytic Leukemia Patients. *Viral Immunol* 2011; 24 (2):165-169.

[31] Cavallo R. The Laboratory of clinical virology in monitoring patients undergoing monoclonal antibody therapy. *Clin Microbiol Infect* 2011; 17: 1781-1785.

[32] O'Brien S, Ravandi F, Riehl T, Wierda W, Huang X, Tarrand J, *et al.* Valganciclovir prevents cytomegalovirus reactivation in patients receiving alemtuzumab-based therapy. *Blood* 2008; 111(4): 1816-1819.

[33] Kaufman M, Rai KR. Review. Alemtuzumab in the up-front setting. *Theraputics and Clinical Risk Management* 2008; 4 (2):459-464.

[34] Fisman DN. Synopsis. Hemophagocytic Syndromes and Infection. *Emerg Infect Dis* 2000; 6 (6): 601-608.

[35] Montillo M, Tedeschi A, Petrizzi VB, Ricci F, Crugnola M, Spriano M, *et al.* An open – label, pilot study of fludarabine, cyclophosphamide, and alemtuzumab in relapsed/refractory patients with B-cell chronic lymphocytic leukemia. *Blood* 2011; 118(15): 4079-4085.

[36] Elter T, Gercheva-Kyuchukova L, Pylypenko H, Robak T, Jaksic B, Rekhtman G, *et al.* Fludarabine plus alemtuzumab versus fludarabine alone in patients with previously treated chronic lymphocytic leukemia: a randomised phase 3 trial. www.thelancet.com/oncology 2011; 12:1204-1213.

[37] Salomon N, Gomez T, Perlman DC, Laya L, Eber C, and Mildvan D. Clinical features and outcome of HIV-related cytomegalovirus Pneumonia. *AIDS* 1997, 11:319-324.

[38] Ayyappan AP, Thomas R, Kurian S, Christopher DJ, and Cherian R. Multiple cavitating masses in an immunocompromised host with rheumatoid arthritis-related interstitial lung disease: an unusual expression of cytomegalovirus pneumonitis. *Brit J Radiol* 2006, 79: e174-e-176.

[39] Moon JH, Kim EA, Lee KS, Kim TS, Jung KJ, and Song JH. Cytomegalovirus Pneumonia High-Resolution CT Findings in Ten Non-AIDS Immunocompromised Patients. *Korean J Radiol* 2000; 1: 73-78.

[40] Vogel MN, Brodoefel H, Hierl T, Beck R, Bethge WA, Claussen CD *et al.* Differences and similarities of cytomegalovirus and pneumocystis Pneumonia in HIV-negative

http://dx.doi.org/10.5772/56141

immunocompromised patients- thin section CT morphology in the early phase of the disease. *Brit J Radiol* 2007; 80:516-523.

[41] Ukarapol N, Chartapisak W, Lertprasertsuk N, Wongsawasdi L, Kattipattanapong V, Singhavejsakul J *et al.* Cytomegalovirus-Associated Manifestations Involving the Digestive Tract in Children With Human Immunodeficiency Virus Infection. *J Pediatr Gastroenterol Nutr* 2002; 35: 669-673.

[42] Ljungman P, Griffiths P, Paya C. Definitions of Cytomegalovirus Infection and Disease in Transplant Recipients. *CID* 2002; 34 (15:1094-1097.

[43] Steininger C. Clinical relevance of cytomegalovirus infection in patients with disorders of the immune system. *Clin Microbiol Infec* 2007; 13: 953–963.

[44] Soderberg-Naucler C. Does cytomegalovirus play a causative role in the development of various inflammatory diseases and cancer? *J Int Med* 2006; 219-246.

[45] Oloomi Z, Moayeri H. Cytomegalovirus Infection-Associated Hemophagocytic Syndrome. *Arch Iranian Med* 2006; 9 (3): 284-287.

[46] Palazzi DL, McClain KL, and Kaplan SL. Major Article. Hemophagocytic Syndrome in Children: An Important Diagnostic Consideration in Fever of Unknown Origin. *CID* 2003; 36: 306-12.

[47] Ponticelli C, and Della Casa Alberighi O. Editorial Reviews. Haemophagocytic syndrome- a life-threatening complication of renal transplantation. *Nephrol Dial Transpl* 2009; 24: 2623-2627.

[48] Raschke RA, and Garcia-Orr R. Original Research. Critical Care. Hemophagocytic Lymphohistiocytosis. A Potentially Underrecognized Association With Systemic Inflammatory Response Syndrome, Severe Sepsis, and Septic Shock in Adults. *Chest* 2011; 140 (4): 933-938.

[49] Núñez Bacarreza JJ, Montiel López L, and Núñez del Prado Alcoreza JR. Elsevier Doyma. Medicina Intensiva. Síndrome hemofagocítico asociado a infección viral por citomegalovirus. *Med Intensiva* 2011; 35 (3): 189-192.

Chapter 4

Cytomegalovirus Infection in Liver Transplantation

Ana Maria Sampaio, Ana Carolina Guardia,
Arlete Milan, Elaine Cristina Ataíde,
Rachel Silveira Bello Stucchi,
Sandra Botelho Cecilia Costa and
Ilka de Fatima Santana Ferreira Boin

Additional information is available at the end of the chapter

http://dx.doi.org/10.5772/56128

1. Introduction

With the global evolution of organ transplantation in humans a new class of patients with special problems related to opportunistic infections after transplantation has appeared [1, 2].Some of these challenges infections with members of the herpesvirus family. Among these viruses, human cytomegalovirus (HCMV) often affects immunocompromised patients, HCMV can be reactivated by immunosuppression and cause significant morbidity and mortality [3,4]. In the postoperative period, HCMV infection can result in serious complications in patients who received grafts by modulating the immune response [5]. However in immunocompetent individuals cytomegalovirus infection can be asymptomatic or cause symptoms similar to infectious mononucleosis syndrome, such as lymphadenopathy, fever, rash, malaise, arthralgia, hepatomegaly and splenomegaly [6].

This chapter presents the main clinical and epidemiological aspects related to cytomegalovirus infection and the importance of detection in liver transplant recipients.

2. Cytomegalovirus history

The discovery of HCMV began in 1881 when the histological effects of infection were observed in the kidney of a newborn child. In 1904, Ribbert identified the causative agent of "cytomegalic inclusion disease", whose name derives from the characteristic cytopathic effect, represented by increases in cell volume and intracellular cytoplasmic inclusions in infected tissues [7]. In 1881 and 1921 similar cell characteristics were reported by Goodpasture and Talbot in a fatal case associated with this virus involving lung, liver and kidney from a newborn child [8].

The first experimental evidence of the likely etiologic agent of "cytomegalic inclusion disease" was proposed by Cole and Kuttner in 1926, when they demonstrated the transmission of the disease in guinea pigs and suggested that this agent possessed characteristics of viral infection and was species-specific. Wolbach and Farber (1932) demonstrated the first evidence that the salivary gland virus was commonly involved and showed typical cytomegalic cells were found in 12% of children. In 1954, using the salivary infection mouse model, Smith isolated the virus in tissue culture [9].

In 1970 study groups were organized to evaluate the impact of infection in immunocompromised people and through this to propose infection control strategies. In the 1980s the control measures of CMV began with antiviral agents and immunological interventions [10].

3. Structure features and replication engine

CMV has an ultrastructure similar to other herpesviruses with four structural elements: an electron-dense core, an icosahedral symmetry capsid, a tegument occupying space between the capsid and an envelope steeped in glycoproteins and membrane proteins [11].

CMV carries a double-stranded DNA containing approximately 240 kb linear bases [12] encoding 33 structural proteins and an indefinite number of non-structural proteins, some of which are antigenic. The genome can be divided into two segments, designated as long component (L) and short (S) defined by repetitive sequence terminals (RT). The CMV has a complex genome due to the acquisitions of host genes and the duplication of viral genes [13]. It is a very thermolabile virus and its average life at 37 ° C is only 45 minutes, totally inactivated at 56 º C for 30 minutes [14].

During natural infection, viral replication can occur in epithelial, endothelial and muscle mesenchymal cells, hepatocytes, granulocytes and macrophages [15, 16]. In vivo studies with cells from immunocompetent and immunosuppressed patients show that CMV can commonly be isolated from polymorphonuclear leukocytes [17], which may represent an important replication site [14,16]. Variants of CMV are found in mice, monkeys and guinea pigs, but these strains are species-specific and do not infect humans [14].

The CMV replication mechanism occurs in three distinct stages, similar to other herpesviruses. The early phase occurs when the virus adheres to the host cell membrane (with the envelope loss and penetration into the cell), in the intermediate phase the gene expression and genome replication occur, and in the late phase, there is the assembly and release of new viral particles [16-18].

The "early" phase begins when surface proteins of the virion adhere to specific protein receptors on the cell surface through non-covalent bonds. The viral particles penetrate by

http://dx.doi.org/10.5772/56128

endocytosis, entering pinocytic vesicles in which the envelope loss process is started, favored by a low pH. The rupture of the vesicles or fusion of the virus with the outer layer of the vesicle membrane deposits the core of the virus in the cell cytoplasm [13].

The intermediate phase lasts 24 hours, characterized by transcription and replication of viral DNA. The first step of viral gene expression is the synthesis of mRNA via host RNA polymerase inside the core. The mRNA is translated by the host ribosomes into early and late viral proteins. The early proteins are enzymes required for viral genome replication [19]. The late proteins include a polymerase replicating the viral genome [13].

In the late phase, viral particles newly formed are grouped together within the capsid and begin the process of budding, during which the nucleocapsid adheres to specific sites of the membrane and interacts with the protein matrix. At this point, a process of evagination occurs and an enveloped particle flows from the membrane surface [13].

4. Transmission and epidemiology

Infection is defined as seroconversion (an increase of 4 times or more in HCMV antibody titer in seronegative or seropositive patients), virus circulation in any body fluid such as urine, nasopharyngeal secretions or blood [7]. CMV infects only the human population and its transmission occurs both horizontally and vertically and may include oropharyngeal secretions, vaginal tears, seminal fluid, breast milk, urine, feces and blood [19]. In adulthood the CMV transmission may occur through heterosexual and homosexual contact, through blood and blood products and through organ transplantation, the latter being an important route of transmission [12,19, 20].

About 80% of the population between late childhood and early adolescence is already infected with CMV [21, 22] and can harbor the virus in various body sites, especially in the salivary glands and different types of leukocytes. With age the increased prevalence of antibodies is common. This may not depend on the geographical area, but the socio-economic status may be important [10, 23- 28]. The seroprevalence of CMV in populations at high socioeconomic level varies from 40% to 60%, increases after infection of early childhood and approximately 10% to 20% of children have their first infection episode before puberty [10]. In lower socioeconomic populations the seroprevalence level is higher, ranging from 80% to 100%. In Brazil, seroprevalence of cytomegalovirus averages 90% in adult populations [28].

5. Clinical manifestations

The clinical course of CMV in immunocompetent individuals may be asymptomatic or may resemble "Mononucleosis Syndrome" presented by persistent fever, myalgia, pharyngitis, lymphadenopathy, sweating and hepatosplenomegaly [10,28-34].

After primary infection, CMV persists in host tissues and may be reactivated to cause disease – usually in children with congenital infection, organ transplant recipients, cancer patients undergoing chemotherapy and patients with HIV disease [7,10,29,35].

Among the complications caused by CMV in transplanted patients increased long-term mortality and worsening graft survival are common [35-37]. Clinical disease caused by CMV is expressed by fever, malaise, myalgia, leukopenia (WBC less than 4.0000/mm^3), increased transaminases (hepatitis), pulmonary (pneumonitis) and/or gastrointestinal (colitis, gastritis, esophagitis) and fever being the most common manifestation, which can also occur with neurological symptomatology compatible with encephalitis but these are rarer [29,38,39].

Clinical disease may reflect

1. Primary infection, when it occurs in patients previously seronegative;
2. Secondary infection occurs when the reactivation of latent infection or superinfection;
3. Tertiary infection by reinfection by other strains of the virus [7].

The source of infection for both primary infection and superinfection is may include graft and blood transfusions. Immunosuppression may cause reactivation of CMV [40]. About two thirds of patients with primary infection are symptomatic, less than 20% in viral reactivation have symptoms and about 40% of reinfected individuals have symptoms attributable to CMV [10]. When primary infection occurs after transplantation the clinical impact is significant [41]. This is most common following allocation of grafts from donors with positive serology to seronegative recipients [42]. Immunosuppressive drugs such as azathioprine and cyclosporine have been implicated in the facilitation of CMV disease [7].

Diagnostic criteria include clinical signs known to be caused by this virus [43,44]. In liver transplant patients with active CMV infection, about 80% will develop clinical manifestations of the disease and the rate may be higher when the recipient is seronegative and a donor is seropositive [44]. CMV infection is an independent risk factor for the development with opportunistic infections, as well as graft rejection [7]. The evidence of viral replication and clinical symptoms in transplant occurs mainly during the 1st to 4th month post-transplant.

The most common clinical manifestations are interstitial pneumonia, esophagitis, gastritis, colitis, retinitis, fever and delayed engraftment in bone marrow transplants [29,45]. During liver transplantation, primary infection tends to be more important as the CMV viremia may be limited to when virus replication is detected in peripheral blood or significant increase of specific antibodies without symptoms or viral syndrome presenting fever equal or greater than 38ºC, malaise, leukopenia, atypical lymphocytosis equal or less than 3-5% and thrombocytopenia [14, 37, 42, 45,46].

Antiviral treatment controls the acute manifestation of the disease in most cases, but may not eradicate the CMV with recurrence reported in 26-31% of solid organ transplant recipients.. [14, 36].

http://dx.doi.org/10.5772/56128

6. Diagnosis

The diagnosis of CMV infection can be done by serology, polymerase chain reaction (PCR), culture and viral antigenemia research. Early diagnosis is important as early treatment of asymptomatic active infection reduces morbidity [24, 31, 46, 47]. The first method of diagnosis used to identify the CMV was exfoliative cytology. This technique revealed the presence of large cells which had inclusions within the core, identified as cytomegalic inclusion. Later methods are more sensitive and specific. These are grouped into seven categories: cytological, histological, virus isolation, serological identification,, **Immunofluorescence, detection of viral antigens** and molecular methods [49, 48]…

Cytopathological techniques: These methods can be performed on tissue and secretions aspirated material [7,8], but have low sensitivity so they currently have little use in clinical practice.

Histological Techniques: A method of detecting inclusions by visualization of typical tissue. The finding of cells with typical inclusions allows often to correlate CMV lesion or dysfunction of the organ studied. Although this method has low sensitivity, it reveals invasive tissue disease [7]. The advantages are low cost, simplicity of use and availability of equipment.

Viral Isolation: CMV can be isolated from various biological materials, such as biological fluids (urine, saliva, blood, cervical secretions, breast milk, tears, semen, feces and washed aspirates organs) and tissue obtained from biopsies or autopsies [49, 50].

Serological methods: The modern serological methods detect the presence of IgM and IgG [51] usually by ELISA. This technique does not detect the virus in early stages of infection, as antibodies are produced by the host only after this phase.

Immunofluorescence (IF): A method that allows an early detection of the virus is immunofluorescence usually using commercially available antibodies.

Detection of Viral Antigens (antigenemia): Antigenemia offers high sensitivity and specificity. It is fast, direct and sensitive, and is considered a quantitative technique for viral load [54, 55]. CMV antigenemia is one of the earlier tests with positive results [17, 25, 51-58] and becomes positive on average 9-18 days before establishment of the disease. It has been widely used for the early detection of active infection in organ transplant recipients [17, 24, 25, 36, 56].

The additional advantage of this method is that results can be expressed quantitatively, allowing observation of the clinical response to treatment [17, 59]. The disadvantage of this technique is the speed needed to process the collected material without loss of sensitivity - 6 to 8 hours [17]. In patients with neutropenia, this test cannot be performed due to low granulocyte count. On this situation, molecular assays are used.

Molecular methods

Polymerase chain reaction-PCR: The qualitative PCR is often the first test to detect asymptomatic subclinical infection, but specific predictive value is low for the diagnosis of HCMV disease. It is not suitable for routine monitoring of patients on treatment [57]...why not???. It is a quick (4-6 hours), specific and extremely sensitive test but false positives may result from contamination during the test run. False negative results can also occur due to presence of inhibitors in the sample [55,60]. The sample type and method of extracting DNA from these samples must be carefully chosen to avoid this [31,61].

Nested PCR (Polymerase Chain Double): Nested PCR (N-PCR) has been used to increase the sensitivity and specificity of simple PCR. Here the product of the first PCR, amplified with a primer pair, is subjected to a new amplification reaction using another pair of primers internal to the first, the product being then detected by agarose gel electrophoresis [62]. Nested PCR technique to diagnose CMV infection produces results consistent with classical culture, reaching 100% specificity and 93% sensitivity in a shorter time frame [63- 66].

Real-time PCR: Real Time PCR amplification (RT PCR) presents high sensitivity and precision. It has been used for the detection and monitoring of viral load. Its sensitivity and specificity are directly related to the choice of "primers" and probes, and the accuracy is determined by the threshold cycle, which is calculated during the exponential phase of the reaction. Formation of a fluorescently labeled product is monitored at each amplification cycle in a single instrument generating quantitative results. [58].

7. Treatment

Ganciclovir has been the "gold standard" for treatment of CMV disease although resistance to this drug has been reported and should be considered in unresponsive patients. Some studies have focused on genotyping of CMV that could indicate samples that were resistant to conventional treatment. Inadequate dosing may reduce clinical efficacy and promote resistance (44)

Antiviral administration is generally initiated in the immediate or early post-transplant period, and continues for 3 to 6 months. Various antiviral drugs have been used, including acyclovir, valaciclovir, intravenous ganciclovir, oral valganciclovir or intravenous (IV) ganciclovir, and valganciclovir. In preventive therapy, laboratory monitoring detects asymptomatic viral replication and antiviral therapy is initiated to prevent progression to clinical disease. For non severe CMV disease, oral valganciclovir (900 mg orally every 12 hr) or IV ganciclovir (5 mg/kg every 12hr) are recommended as first-line treatment. Renal function should be monitored frequently during treatment, with estimated or measured glomerular filtration rate. Optimal length of treatment should be achieved by monitoring weekly viral loads and treating until one or two consecutive negative samples are obtained, but not shorter than 2 weeks. Duration should reflect the likelihood of recurrent CMV infection. In cases of serious disease and in tissue-invasive disease without viremia, longer treatment periods with clinical monitoring of the specific disease manifestation are recommended. In cases of recurrent CMV disease, prophylaxis after retreatment may need to be prolonged. [44].

http://dx.doi.org/10.5772/56128

8. Transplantation

CMV seroprevalence is high in developing countries such as Brazil, so most of the patients and/or donors is CMV IgG positive. The techniques chosen for the laboratorial monitoring in our service after liver transplantation are antigenemia and Nested-PCR (N-PCR). These techniques detect the active viral replication and minimize the damage of the disease caused by CMV (see Section **xy**).

We diagnose active infection from one positive result by antigenemia, or two positive N-PCR findings over an interval equal or smaller than 30 days. As antigenemia can detect CMV a few days to one week before the appearance of the symptoms, the Ganciclovir is initiated after the detection of a positive cell even without clinical symptoms if the patient presents IgG negative and the donor presents IgG positive. Patients are monitored while in hospital and after discharge following a protocol: weekly from the first to the second month, fortnightly in the third-fourth months and monthly until six months. After this period the antigenemia or N-PCR is performed only if there is a suggestive clinical diagnosis of CMV infection. The assessment of antigenemia also provides an estimate of viral load that is useful in the differentiation of CMV disease from other complications. Thus we evaluate the efficacy of antiviral therapy and have capacity to detect drug resistance.

CMV is frequently detected in our patients after liver transplantation [24,25,30,31]. Detection of N-PCR and antigenemia are useful markers for active infection [30,31].The rates of CMV found in our groups are similar to other services [24,25,30-32].

We also observed that symptomatic CMV infection occurs during the first three months after transplantation. We consider that this high incidence of symptomatic CMV infection is due to the high prevalence of the virus in Brazilian population. The mean time for initial detection CMV is around 29 days following transplantation (range: 0-99 days) [30]..

In our service, CMV DNA diagnosed in pretransplantation graft biopsy specimens remained positive posttransplantation on graft biopsies. This common complication negatively influences liver transplantation outcomes and is a risk factor to develop acute cellular rejection episodes [67].Ganciclovir prophylaxis for CMV is not performed at our institution unless the patient is preoperative negative IgG and the donor is CMV positive. Prophylaxis is performed only for herpes simplex type 1 with Acyclovir.

Another relevant issue at our service is opportunistic infections, which are often seen in patients at risk for CMV and have been recognized by our staff as a significant risk factor for graft failure and death [24]. Active CMV infection may increase the risk of bacterial, fungal, viral, and others, as well as post-transplant lymphoproliferative disease. [31] This includes co-infections by other viruses of the same family (HHV-6, HHV-7) [24,32].

The clinical impact of CMV-infected patients observed by our team [24] shows that it is extremely important to follow up these patients. These data have helped the medical staff making therapeutic strategies to minimize risks caused by this betaherpesvirus.

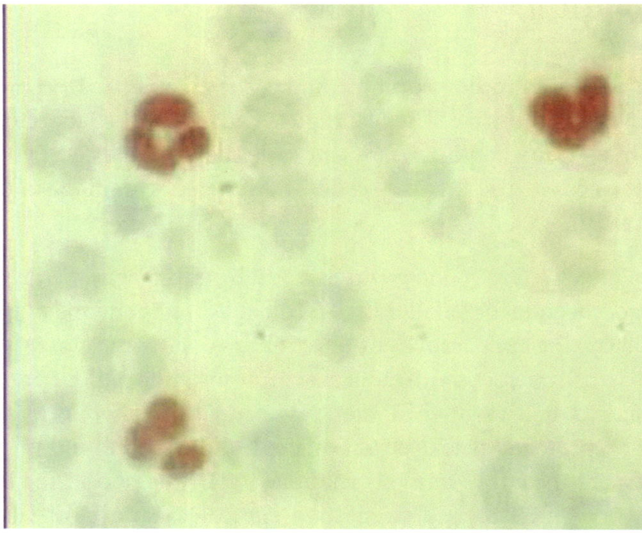

Figure 1. Nuclei of neutrophils stained in brown indicating positive pp65-atigenemia (counterstained with Harris's hematoxylin). Mouse C10 and C11 monoclonal antibodies against pp65-matrix CMV antigen and rabbit anti-mouse Ig horseradish peroxidase conjugate. The reaction was revealed by hydrogen peroxide and amino-ethyl-carbazole[24]

Virus	Synonym	Subfamily	Abbreviation
Human Herpesvirus-1	Herpes simplex-1	||	HSV-1/HHV-1
Human Herpesvirus -2	Herpes simplex-2	||	HSV-2/HHV-2
Human Herpesvirus -3	Varicella-zoster	||	VZV/HHV-3
Human Herpesvirus -4	Epstein-Barr	||	EBV/HSV-4
Human Herpesvirus -5	Cytomegalovirus	||	HCMV/CMV/HHV-5
Human Herpesvirus -6	None	||	HHV-6
Human Herpesvirus -7	None	||	HHV-7
Human Herpesvirus -8	None	||	KSHV/HHV-8

Table 1. Complete list of human herpesvirus

9. Conclusion

Few patients remain free of betaherpesvirus after liver transplantation. Active CMV infection is common especially in the first weeks after grafting. We believe it is important to continue monitoring CMV infection after transplantation, especially when the prevalence in the general population is high.

http://dx.doi.org/10.5772/56128

Acknowledgements

Biologist Eliana Duarte Quizini Bueno

This study received financial support from Coordenação de Aperfeiçoamento de Pessoal de Nível Superior (CAPES).

Author details

Ana Maria Sampaio[1], Ana Carolina Guardia[1], Arlete Milan[2], Elaine Cristina Ataíde[1], Rachel Silveira Bello Stucchi[2], Sandra Botelho Cecilia Costa[2] and Ilka de Fatima Santana Ferreira Boin[1*]

*Address all correspondence to: ilkaboin@yahoo.com

1 Department of Surgery - Liver Transplant Unit of the State University of Campinas, Brazil

2 Department of Clinical Medicine - Liver Transplantation Unit, State University of Campinas, Brazil

References

[1] Levinson, W, & Jawetz, E. Medical microbiology & immunology: examination and board review 6th ed. New York: Lange Medical Books/McGraw-Hill (2000). Part. IV., 206-282.

[2] Tong CYWBakran A, Willians H, Cheung CY, Peiris JSM. Association of human herpes virus 7 with CMV disease in renal transplant recipients. Transplantation (2000). , 70-213.

[3] Guo, Z, Chen, H. R, Liu, X. D, Bian, J. M, He, X. F, Lou, J. X, et al. Clinical analysis of cytomegalovirus infection after allogeneic hematopoietic stem cell transplantation Zhong Shi Yan Xue Ye Xue Za Zhi (2012). , 20(4), 971-4.

[4] Lautenschlager, I, Halme, L, Hockerstedt, K, Krogerus, L, & Taskinen, E. Cytomegalovirus infection of the Liver Transplant: Virological, Histological, Immunological, and Clinical Observations. Transpl Infect Dis (2006). , 8-21.

[5] Weigand, K, Schnitzler, P, Schimidt, J, Chahoud, F, Gotthardt, D, Schemmer, P, et al. Cytomegalovirus Infection After Liver Transplantation Incidence, Risks, And Benefits of Prophylaxis. Transplant Proc (2010). , 42-2634.

[6] Schroeder, R, Michelon, T, Fagundes, I, Bortolotto, A, Lammerhirt, E, Oliveira, J, et al. Cytomegalovirus disease latent and active infection rates during the first trimester after kidney transplantation. Transplant Proc (2004). , 36, 896-8.

[7] Maya TC; Azulay DRInfecção pelo Citomegalovirus. In: Lupi O; Silva AS; Pereira Jr. Herpes- Clinica, Diagnóstico e Tratamento, 1° Ed., Medsi Editora Médica e Científica (2000). , 8-135.

[8] Drew, W. L. Diagnosis of cytomegalovirus infection. Rev Infect Dis (1988). , 3-468.

[9] Smith, I. L, Cherrington, J. M, Jiles, R. E, Fuller, M. D, Freeman, W. R, & Spector, S. A. High-level resistance of cytomegalovirus to ganciclovir is associated with alterations in both the UL97 and DNA polymerase genes. J Infect Dis (1997). , 176(1), 69-77.

[10] Costa SCBInfecção por citomegalovirus (CMV); epidemiologia, diagnóstico e tratamento. Rev Bras Clín Ter (1999). , 18-28.

[11] Braun, D. L, Dominguez, G, & Pellet, P. E. Human Herpesvirus 6. Clinic Microbiol Review (1997). , 10-521.

[12] Brennan, D. C. *Cytomegalovirus* in Renal Transplantation. J Am Soc Nephrology (2001). , 12-848.

[13] Levinson, W, & Jawetz, E. Medical Microbiology & Immunology: Examination & Board Review 6th ed. New York: Lange Medical Books/McGraw-Hill (2000). , 206-282.

[14] Rowshani, A. T. Clinical and immunologic aspects of cytomegalovirus infection in solid organ transplant recipients. Transplantation (2005). , 79, 381-386.

[15] Smith, V. V, Williams, A. J, Novelli, V, & Malone, M. Extensive enteric leiomyolysis due to cytomegalovirus enterocolitis in vertically acquired human immunodeficiency virus infection in infants. Pediatr Dev Pathol (2000). , 3(6), 591-6.

[16] Gerna, G, Percivalle, E, Baldanti, F, Sozzani, S, Lanzarini, P, Genin, I, et al. Human cytomegalovirus replicates abortively in polymorphonuclear leukocytes after transfer from infected endothelial cells via transient microfusion events. J Virol (2000). , 74, 5629-5638.

[17] Bonon SHAMenoni SMF, Rossi CL, Souza CA, Costa SCB. Surveillance of cytomegalovirus infection in hematopoietic stem cell transplantation patients. J Infection (2005). , 50, 130-13.

[18] Santos RLBPropriedades Gerais dos Herpesvírus. In: Lupi A, Silva AS, Pereira JR, AC.- Herpes Clín Diag Trat 1ª edição, Medsi Editora Médica e Científica Ltda (2000). , 10-79.

[19] Bresnahan, W. A, & Shenk, T. A Subset of viral transcripts package within human cytomegalovirus particles. *Science* (2000).

[20] Drago, F, Aragone, M. G, Luagni, C, & Rebora, A. Cytomegalovirus Infection in normal and immunocompromised humans. Dermatology (2000). , 200-189.

[21] Almeida, L, Azevedo, B, Amaku, R S, & Massad, M. E. *Cytomegalovirus* seroepidemiology in an urban community of são paulo, Brazil. Rev Saúde Pública (2001). , 35(2), 124-129.

[22] Gupteat, M, Diaz-mitoma, F, Feber, J, Shaw, L, Forget, C, & Filler, G. Tissue HHV6 and HHV7 determination in pediatric solid organ recipients- a Pilot Study. Ped Transplant (2003). , 7, 458-463.

[23] Pannuti, C. S, & Vilas, B. Neto LSVA, Ângelo MJO, Sabbada E. Detecção de anticorpos IgM nas interações primárias e secundárias pelo citomegalovirus em pacientes submetidos a transplante renal. Inst Med Trop (1987). , 29, 317-322.

[24] Sampaio, A. M, Thomasini, R. L, Guardia, A. C, Stucchi, R. S, Rossi, C. L, Costa, S. C, et al. Cytomegalovirus, human herpesvirus-6, and human herpesvirus-7 in adult liver transplant recipients: diagnosis based on antigenemia. Transplant Proc (2011). , 434, 1357-9.

[25] Milan, A, Sampaio, A. M, Guardia, A. C, Pavan, C. R, Andrade, P. D, Bonon, S. H, et al. Monitoring and detection of cytomegalovirus in liver transplant recipients. Transplant Proc (2011). , 43, 1360-1.

[26] Miller, C. S, Avdiushko, S. A, Kryscio, R. J, Danaher, R. J, & Jacob, R. J. Effect of prophylactic valaciclovir on the presence of human herpesvirus dna in saliva healthy individuals after dental treatment. J Clin Microbiol (2005). , 5, 2173-80.

[27] Crumpacker, C. S, & Wadhwa, S. Cytomegalovirus. In: Mandell GL, Bennett JE, Dolin R. Principles and Practice of Infectious Disease. 6 ed. Philadelphia: Elsevier Inc (2005). , 1786-96.

[28] Aquino, V. H, & Figueiredo, L. M. Cytomegalovirus Infection in renal transplant recipients diagnosed by Nested-PCR. Braz J Med (2001). , 34(2), 93-101.

[29] Razonable, R. R, & Paya, C. V. Infections and allograft rejection- Intertwined complications of organ transplantation. Swiss Med Wkly (2005). , 135-39.

[30] Costa, F. A, Soki, M. N, & Andrade, P. D. Bonon SHA, Thomasini RL, Sampaio AM, et al. Simultaneous monitoring of cmv and human herpesvirus 6 infections and diseases in liver transplant patients: one-year follow-up. Clinics (2011). , 66, 949-53.

[31] Thomasini, R. L, Sampaio, A. M, Bonon, S. H, Boin, I. F, Leonardi, L. S, Leonardi, M, et al. Detection and monitoring of human herpesvirus 7 in adult liver transplant patients: impact on clinical course and association with cytomegalovirus. Transplant Proc (2007). , 39, 1537-9.

[32] Guardia, A. C, Stucchi, R. S, Sampaio, A. M, Milan, A, Costa, S. C, Pavan, C. R, et al. human herpesvirus 6 in donor biopsies associated with the incidence of clinical cyto-

megalovirus disease and hepatitis c virus recurrence. Int J Infect Dis (2011). , 16, 124-9.

[33] Sebeková, K, Feber, J, Carpenter, B, Shaw, L, Karnauchow, T, Diaz-mitoma, F, et al. Tissue viral dna is associated with chronic allograft nephropathy (2005)., 95, 598-603.

[34] Pannuti, C. S. Citomegalia. In: Ferreira, A. W.; Ávila, S.L.M. eds. Diagnóstico Laboratorial das principais Doenças Infecciosas e Autoimunes, 2ª. Edição, Editora Guanabara Koogan (2001)., 5-68.

[35] Linhares, L, Sanclemente, G, Cervera, C, Hoyo, I, Cofán, F, Ricart, M. J, et al. Influence of cytomegalovirus disease in outcome of solid organ transplant patients. Transplant Proc (2011)., 43, 2145-2148.

[36] Sampathkumar, P, & Paya, C. V. Management of cytomegalovirus infection after liver transplantation. Liver Transpl (2000)., 6(2), 144-156.

[37] Angelis, M, Cooper, J, & Freeman, R. B. Impact of donor infections on outcome of orthotopic liver transplantation (2003)., 451-462.

[38] Ljungman, P, Griffiths, P, & Paya, C. Definition of cytomegalovirus infection and disease in transplant recipients. Clin Infect Dis (2002).

[39] Humar, A, Kumar, D, Gray, M, Moussa, G, Venkataraman, S, Kumar, R, & Tipples, G. A. A Prospective assessment of cytomegalovirus immune evasion gene transcription profiles in transplant patients with cytomegalovirus infection. Transplantation (2007)., 83(9), 1200-6.

[40] Van Der MeerJtm Drew.; Bowden RA.; Galasso Gl.; Griffiths PD.; Jabs DA; et al. Summary of the international consensus symposium on advances in the diagnosis, treatment and prophylaxis of cytomegalovirus infection. Antiviral Res (1996). , 32, 119-140.

[41] Singh, N, Wannstedt, C, Keyes, L, Wagener, M. M, Vera, M, Cacciarelli, T. V, et al. Impact of evolving trends in recipient and donor characteristics on cytomegalovirus infection in liver transplant recipients. Transplantation (2004)., 77, 106-10.

[42] Freeman, R. B. Risk factors for cytomegalovirus viremia and disease developing after prophylaxis in high-risk solid-organ transplant recipients. Transplantation (2004). , 78, 1765-1773.

[43] Mustafa, M. M. Cytomegalovirus infection and disease in the immunocompromised host. The Ped Inf Dis J (1994)., 13, 249-259.

[44] Kotton, C. N, Humar, A, Caliendo, A. M, Emery, V, Lautenschlager, I, Lazzarotto, T, et al. Transplantation Society International CMV Consensus Group. International consensus guidelines on the management of cytomegalovirus in solid organ transplantation. Transplantation (2010)., 89, 779-95.

[45] Seehofer, D, et al. CMV hepatitis after liver transplantation: incidence, clinical course, and long-term follow-up. Liver Transpl (2002).

[46] Hoppe, L, Bressane, R, Lago, L. S, Schiavo, F. L, & Mar, K. L. Castisani CPC. Risk factors associated with cytomegalovirus-positive antigenemia in orthotopic liver transplant patients. Transplant Proc (2004)., 36, 961-963.

[47] Lautenschlager, J, Lappalainen, M, Linnavuori, K, Suni, J, & Hockerstedt, K. CMV infection is usually associated with concurrent HHV-6 and HHV-7 antigenemia in liver transplant Patients. J Clin Virol (2002)., 25-57.

[48] Chou, S. Newer methods for diagnosis of cytomegalovirus infection. Rev Infect Dis (1990).

[49] Lautenschlager, I, Linnavuori, K, Lappalainen, M, Suni, J, & Höckerstedt, K. HHV-6 reactivation is often associated with CMV infection in liver transplant patients. Transpl Int (2000)., 131-351.

[50] Ho, M. Cytomegalovirus: Biology and infection. Plen Publis Corp (1991)., 1-440.

[51] Biganzoli, P, Ferreyra, L, Sicilia, P, Carabajal, C, Frattari, S, Littvik, A, et al. IgG Subclasses and DNA detection of HHV-6 and HHV-7 in healthy individuals. J Med Virol (2010)., 82, 1679-83.

[52] Rasmussen, L, Kelsall, D, Nelson, R, Carney, W, Hirsch, M, Winston, D, et al. Virus-specific IgG and IgM antibodies in normal and immunocompromised subjects infected with cytomegalovirus. J Infect Dis (1982)., 145(2), 191-9.

[53] Chantlynne, L. G, & Ablashi, D. V. Seroepidemiology of Kaposi's sarcoma-associated herpesvirus (KSHV). Semin Cancer Biol (1999).

[54] Van Den Berg APKlompmaker IJ, Haagsma EB, Scolten-Sampson A, Bijlevel CMA; Schirm J, et al. Antigenemia in the diagnosis and monitoring of active cytomegalovirus infection after liver transplantation. J Infect Dis (1991)., 164, 265-270.

[55] The, T. H, Van Der Ploeg, M, Van Der Berg, A. P, Vlieger, A. M, et al. Direct detection of cytomegalovirus in peripheral blood leukocytes: a review of the antigenemia assay and polymerase chain reaction. Transplantation (1992)., 54, 193-198.

[56] Schroeder, R, Michelon, T, Fagundes, I, et al. Antigenemia for Cytomegalovirus in renal transplantation: choosing a cutoff for the diagnosis criteria in cytomegalovirus disease. Transplant Proc (2005)., 37, 2781-2783.

[57] Amorim, M. L, Cabeda, J. M, Seca, R, Mendes, A. C, Castro, A. P, & Amorim, J. M. CMV infection of liver transplant recipients: comparison of antigenemia and molecular biology assays. BMC Infect Dis (2001).

[58] Bordils, A, Plumed, J. S, Ramos, D, Beneyto, I, Mascarós, V, Molina, J. M, et al. comparison of quantitative pcr and antigenemia in cytomegalovirus infection in renal transplant recipients. Transplant Proc (2005)., 37, 3756-9.

[59] Lianghui, G, Shusen, Z, Tinoba, L, Yan, S, Welling, W, & Anwei, L. Deferred versus prophylactic therapy with ganciclovir for cytomegalovirus in allograft liver transplantation. Transplant Proc (2004). , 36, 1502-1505.

[60] Piiparinen, H, Höckerstedt, K, Grönhagen-riska, C, & Lautenschlager, I. Comparison of two quantitative CMV PCR tests, Cobas Amplicor CMV monitor and taqman assay, and assay in the determination of viral loads from peripheral blood of organ transplant patients. J Clin Virol (2004). , 65.

[61] Peigo, M. F, Thomasini, R. L, Puglia, A. L, Costa, S. C, Bonon, S. H, Boin, I. F, et al. Human herpesvirus-7 in brazilian liver transplant recipients. a follow-op comparison between molecular and immunological assays. Transplant Infect Dis (2009). , 11, 497-502.

[62] Abecassis, M. M, Koffron, A. J, Buckingham, M, Kaufman, D. B, Fryer, J. P, Stuart, J, et al. Role of PCR in the diagnosis and management of cmv in solid organ recipients. what is the predictive value for development of disease and should pcr be used to guide antiviral therapy. Transplant Proc (1997).

[63] Olive, D. M, et al. Mufti S, Simsek M, Fayez H, al Nakib W. Direct Detection of Human Cytomegalovirus in Urine Specimens From Renal Transplant Patients Following Polymerase Chain Reaction Amplification. J Med Virol (1989). , 29(4), 232-7.

[64] Costa, F. A, Soki, M. N, & Andrade, P. D. Bonon SHA, Thomasini RL, Sampaio AM, et al. Simultaneous monitoring of CMV and human herpesvirus 6 infections and diseases in liver transplant patients: one-year follow-up. Clinics (2011). , 66, 949-53.

[65] Evans, M. J, Edwards-spring, Y, Myers, J, Wendt, A, Povinelli, D, Amsterdam, D, et al. Polymerase chain reaction assays for the detection of cytomegalovirus in organ and bone marrow transplant recipients. Immunol Invest (1997).

[66] Gerna, G, Zavattoni, M, Percivalle, E, Zella, D, Torsellini, M, & Revello, M. G. Diagnosis of human cytomegalovirus infections in the immunocompromised host. Clin Diagn Virol (1996).

[67] Guardia-silva, A. C, Stucchi, R. S, Sampaio, A. M, Milan, A, Costa, S. C, & Boin, I. F. Detection of cytomegalovirus and human herpesvirus-6 DNA in liver biopsy specimens and their correlation with rejection after liver transplantation. Transplant Proc. (2012). , 44(8), 2441-4.

Chapter 5

The Footprint of CMV Infection May Last a Lifetime

Patricia Price

Additional information is available at the end of the chapter

http://dx.doi.org/10.5772/54798

1. Introduction

Cytomegalovirus (CMV) is a β-herpesvirus able to replicate in fibroblasts, endothelial cells and monocytes [1]. CMV infection is usually asymptomatic, but causes a mononucleosis-like illness in some individuals. CMV disease can manifest as a syndrome or as an acute infection of an organ or tissue. CMV syndrome is characterized by fever, leukopenia, hepato-splenomegaly, myalgias and occasionally pneumonitis. Sites of acute CMV infection include brain, heart, kidneys, liver and eyes. CMV colitis and CMV enteritis are manifestations of CMV disease in solid organ transplant recipients, bone marrow transplant recipients and HIV patients [2]. CMV retinitis was a common AIDS-defining illness before antiretroviral therapy (ART) became available, and remains a significant cause of blindness in HIV patients in the developing world [3]

In considering the role of CMV in human health, many studies have overlooked the fact that 50-90% of all populations are seropositive. As the virus has the capacity of latency and is known to be reactivated by "stress" (immunosuppression), it is likely that most people harbour latent virus [2]. Much of literature related to CMV is derived from studies of laboratory mice infected with a related virus Murine Cytomegalovirus (MCMV), which shares a similar genomic organisation and some sequence homology with human CMV. It is promoted as a useful model to study host-interaction because it shares similar in-vivo properties to human CMV after infection. Differences in the susceptibility of inbred strains of laboratory mice to MCMV infection has allowed several mechanisms of virological control to be characterised [4, 5], but there are several areas where extrapolation to human CMV is problematic.

1. CMV has over 200 reading frames with potential to encode proteins [1].Of the proteins characterised, many are redundant for viral replication *in vitro*. These include homologues of host genes "picked up" since mice and humans diverged during mammalian evolution. If we assume that such genes are retained because they confer a survival advantage, then

the pathogenic pathways initiated by the murine and human viruses must be subtly different. This has been demonstrated with CMV-encoded chemokines [6].

2. Susceptibility to murine CMV is MHC (murine *H-2*) dependent. This is evident in cultured cells and immunodeficient hosts so it is not related to CD8+ T-cell responses. Rather some *H-2* Class I proteins appear to act as a cell surface receptor. There is no evidence that human HLA proteins have this role [7].

3. Without external immunosuppression, adult laboratory mice of susceptible strains can readily be infected with murine CMV at a dose that destroys their spleen and other organs, and may cause death [4].This is not seen in people, but has been used in many studies to examine immune responses to CMV.

4. *In vitro* infection of monocytes, macrophages and dendritic cells with murine CMV [8, 9] creates cells which remain intact but selectively loose secondary functions. This is interesting but not an important mode of immunoregulation, as only a small percentage of cells of these lineages are infected in patients or more resistant mice.

To avoid translational issues between studies of MCMV in mice and HCMV in humans, we need to look more closely at people infected with CMV. This must include primary disease and the effects of long term asymptomatic CMV infection in immune competent hosts. A lesson that we can take from MCMV is the effects on multiple cells and organs, including the adrenals, pancreas and salivary glands [4, 5, 10, 11]. Sensitive PCR-based viral load assays are now available, but these are only routinely applied to blood, urine or saliva of patients at risk of acute disease. There is little probability of detecting latent CMV. Here we present a tool to evaluate the lifetime effects of CMV on human health - the footprint of CMV. We also summarise evidence that natural killer (NK) cells may regulate the footprint of CMV. The likely impact in HIV patients is presented as Figure 1.

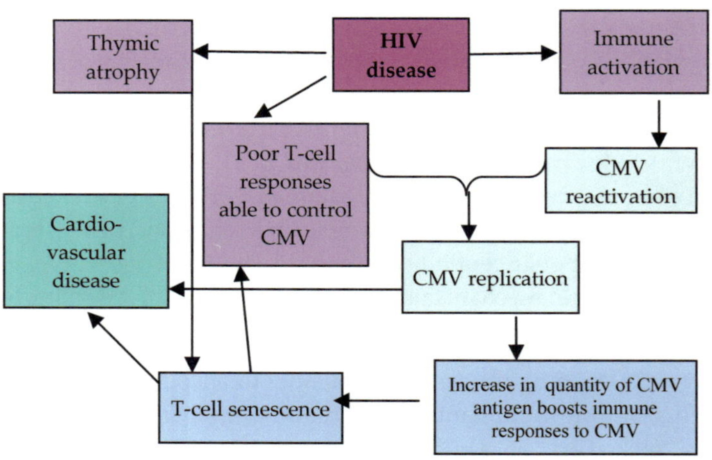

Figure 1. HIV disease has several avenues to enhance the footprint of CMV and thereby promote cardiovascular disease.

http://dx.doi.org/10.5772/54798

2. Immune control of CMV

T-cell and antibody responses may reflect CMV replication rather than protect against it. CD8+ T-cell responses to CMV can be assessed by IFNγ ELISpot or using tetramers or pentamers that mark cells reacting with a particular CMV peptide presented by a particular HLA molecule (usually HLA-A2). Gamadia *et al* [12]reported that frequencies of CMV-specific $CD8^+$ T-cells were significantly higher in immunosuppressed transplant recipients than in healthy donors, suggesting that these responses may reflect exposure rather than protection. This is consistent with evidence that CMV encodes proteins that down regulate T-cell recognition of infected cells, and thus evade immune detection. This includes the degradation of HLA class I and II molecules by unique short (US) proteins and disruption of antigen processing by an infected antigen-presenting cell [13].CMV-specific cells predominantly have an effector-memory or senescent phenotype ($CD45R0^+CD27^-CCR7^-$ or $CD45RA^+CD27^-CCR7^-$, resp.). Subsequent studies suggest that a rapid $CD4^+$ T-cell response was also essential to avoid symptomatic primary CMV infection in renal transplant recipients [14], but the cells critical for the maintenance of latency have not been identified.

Extensive studies of MCMV infection in laboratory mice have mapped protective NK cell-mediated responses to the Ly49 gene cluster [equivalent to human Killer Cell Immunoglobulin-like receptor (KIR) genes]. Mouse strains have distinct Ly49 gene repertoires, which correlate with resistance to MCMV [15]. The activating receptor Ly49H is implicated in protection, and several members of the Ly49 family interact with MCMV encoded proteins [16]. In mice without a protective NK response (eg: through Ly49H), MCMV infections are eventually controlled by T-cells. $CD4^+$ T-cells are needed to control MCMV persistence in the salivary gland [17]. $CD8^+$ T-cells recognising immediate early (IE) epitopes are also implicated in control of reactivated MCMV, where frequent boosting expands specific $CD8^+$ T-cell clones. MCMV encodes genes able to regulate MHC class I expression, demonstrating an evolutionary impetus to avoid $CD8^+$ T-cell responses. Critical epitopes and *H-2* loci initiating protective $CD8^+$ T-cell responses have been identified, but it is a limitation that all studies use laboratory strains of MCMV rather than primary isolates [18]. This highlights the need to study human CMV disease.

Direct evidence that NK cells can control CMV in humans is available from a study of a congenitally T-cell deficient child with acute CMV infection and a 10-fold expansion of NK cells with restricted receptor diversity. Acute illness resolved and NK cells returned to normal levels with clearance of plasma CMV DNA [19].This fits teleological and genetic evidence that NK cells control CMV. Human and mouse CMV diverged with their host species and have independently evolved proteins able to subvert protective NK responses [20]. This includes homologues of HLA-G (UL18) and HLA-E signal peptide (UL40), which interact with NK inhibitory receptors (LIR-1 and NKG2C, resp.) (Reviewed in[21]) In support of a role for NK cells in CMV and HIV disease, we showed that heterozygous carriage of allele 2 at LIR-1 (rs1061680; LILRB1 I142T) associated with CMV disease and nadir $CD4^+$ T-cell counts [22].

A role for NK cells in the control of CMV is also consistent with evidence that carriage of more genes for activating KIR receptors protects against CMV reactivation in immunosuppressed renal [23, 24] and bone marrow [25, 26] transplant patients. KIR receptors in man comprise both inhibitory and activating members (as do Ly49 genes in mice). The ligands for most inhibitory KIR are allelic epitopes of the classical class I HLA proteins (reviewed in[27]). In contrast, ligands for most of the activating KIR are unknown. An exception is KIR2DS1, which interacts with HLA-C2. [28, 29]. Several groups have attempted to identify the CMV-protective KIR gene, but this is complicated by linkage disequilibrium in the KIR gene complex. Inhibition of NK killing of fibroblasts infected by CMV has been demonstrated by several groups [30].This study implicated UL18 but this may depend on the NK donor's genotype. Although the roles of specific NK receptors in CMV disease are unclear, increased expression of LIR-1 [31, 32] and/or NKG2C [33, 34] is a consequence (footprint) of CMV replication. This has potential as a tool to assess a history of CMV reactivation.

3. CMV has a footprint in healthy aging and cardiovascular disease

Associations between CMV and vasculopathy have been described since 1987 [35] and attributed to immunopathological events initiated by viral replication. Our studies of MCMV in inbred mice showed that susceptible BALB/c mice develop myocarditis in which CD8+ T-cells accumulate in the myocardium and persist for 12 months despite clearance of viral antigen by day 3 [36]. In C57BL/6 mice have a protective NK response [5] and display only mild resolving myocarditis. To evaluate the evidence available in patients requires consideration of the underlying mechanisms.

Inflammation and activation of immune cells features throughout atherogenic plaque formation, which is the principle condition of cardiovascular disease (CVD). Pathogenesis of atherosclerotic plaques on vessel walls begins with acute inflammation resulting in endothelium dysfunction [37]. Many life-style risk factors can reduce the integrity of endothelium. The accumulation of low density lipoproteins (LDL) in intimal space by diffusion and its oxidation can cause endothelial cell injury and inflammation [38]. Secretion of vascular cell adhesion molecule-1 (VCAM-1) and up-regulation of selectins and integrins facilitates leukocyte adhesion to vessel walls. Inflammatory cytokines such as IL-1 and TNF-α induce expression of chemokines (eg: CCL2, CXCL8, CX3CL1) by endothelial cells, recruiting T-cells and monocytes and facilitating their transmigration into the intimal space. Monocytes internalize LDL and differentiate into macrophages which promote inflammation and leukocyte migration into developing plaques by secretion of CX3CL1/CX3CR1, interferon-γ (IFNγ) and CCL2 [39, 40] and generation of reactive oxygen species [41]. Hyperlipidemia, macrophage death and consequential irregular surfaces of vessel endothelium promote growth of the atherosclerotic lesion. Smooth muscle cells migrate from the media to intimal space aided by lytic enzymes. This contributes to plaque instability [39]. Smooth muscle cells proliferate in intimal space and also adhere to monocytes [42], thickening arterial walls and occluding the vessel. Rupture of the plaque can result in infarction. Myocardial infarcts (MI) refer to rupture of plaque in the coronary artery. The carotid artery is also a frequent site of plaque formation and thickness of the intima at this site can indicate clinical and sub-clinical CVD [43].

Active CMV infection has been associated with the onset of autoimmune disorders in transplant patients and healthy donors. The development of autoimmune antibodies following reactivation of CMV in transplant patients has been linked to graft versus host disease and graft rejection. Hypergammaglobulinemia and autoantibody production can also be a feature of CMV-induced mononucleosis. There have been several case reports of healthy individuals developing acute CMV infection preceding vasculitis or encephalitis. In a case of encephalitis, treatment of active CMV with valganciclovir resolved symptoms, but CMV-specific CD4+ and CD8+ T-cells remained 10 months after disease onset [44-]. The development of autoimmune vasculitis, systemic lupus erythematosus, sclerodoma and necrotizing vasculitis have been associated with CMV replication [46]. Anti-phospholipid antibodies have been shown to activate endothelial cells and CMV transcription [47], suggesting a feedback amplification loop.

CMV seropositivity has been correlated with a greater risk of all-cause mortality in the elderly [48-]. Although it is rare for CMV to be identified as the primary cause of death, CMV prevalence in the older population can be as high as 100% [52]. An in-depth study following Latinos aged 60-101 years for a period of 9 years (n=1,468) showed that those with high CMV antibody titres were 1.43 times more likely to die and had 1.35 times greater risk of CVD-associated mortality than those with low CMV antibody titres [51]. 96% of the participants were CMV seropositive. Factors significantly ($p<0.05$) associated with mortality included age, female gender, low education level and levels of inflammatory markers (TNF, IL-6, C-reactive protein). Elderly CMV-seropositive patients respond less well to seasonal influenza vaccination than those with low or negative CMV seropositivity [50, 53]. This suggests dysfunction of the immune system and could account for the increased risk of all-cause mortality.

In older CMV-seropositive adults, up to 23% of the T-cell population can be CMV-specific. For example, NLV peptide-specific CD8+ T-cells alone comprised a median 3% (range = 0.4-5.6%) of CD8+ T-cells in donors aged 90 [89-96] years. CMV-specific T-cells are generally CD28-negative(an immunosenescent phenotype also associated with expression of CD57 and shortened telomeres) and have limited proliferative potential, but may produce IFNγ. Their accumulation correlates with immunologic aging or "immunosenescence" evident in the entire T-cell population assayed *ex vivo* [54-].The accumulation of senescent CMV-reactive T-cells was greatest in frail and institutionalized elderly donors [58].Repeated sub-clinical CMV infections may expand CMV-specific T-cells clones until they suppress homeostatic expansion of other T-cells. Alternatively the expanded clones of CMV-reactive cells may bias the population and dilute cells of other specificities - explaining why EBV-reactive T-cells do not show a senescent phenotype [54].

However chronic CMV reactivation may have wider consequences than just an aging immune system. CMV infects endothelial cells in acute stages of infection and it is proposed they could also be a site of latent infection [59, 60]. Studies of murine CMV in mice have identified endothelial cells as a site of viral latency [61], whilst several studies demonstrated human CMV in arterial walls of atherosclerotic and non-atherosclerotic patients [62, 63]. A study of tissues removed during surgery for abdominal aortic aneurysm associated the presence of CMV DNA in smooth muscle cells with expression of inflammatory mediators and implicated CMV in the pathology [64]. Accordingly higher CMV antibody titres are associated with increased diastolic and systolic blood pressure in young men [65] and CMV seropositivity is more frequent in coronary artery disease requiring surgery[66]. Increased expression of LIR-1 on NK cells (a footprint of CMV) is also associated with atherosclerosis [67].Stronger T-cell responses to CMV also associate with severe cardiovascular changes seen in HIV patients [68].

The chemokine, fractalkine (CX3CL1) and its receptor CX3CR1 are membrane-bound proteins. CX3CL1 can be cleaved from a cell surface through TNFα signal pathways to mediate attraction and then firm adhesion of lymphocytes expressing CX3CR1 to endothelium. T-lymphocytes and monocytes express CX3CR1, whilst monocytes, endothelial cells and smooth muscle cells can be induced to express CX3CL1 by TNFα, IFNγ, IL-1 and LPS [37, 69, 70].CX3CR1 is found in atherosclerotic plaques and its role in plaque formation and mediation by inflammation is of interest in the management of CVD [69]. An *in vitro* system co-coculturing CMV infected endothelial cells and peripheral blood mononuclear cells established the principle that CMV specific CD4+ T-cells can induce CX3CL1 production in CMV infected endothelial cells. CX3CL1 aids the ingress of monocytes and NK cells which are capable of killing the CMV infected endothelial cell [71].

Monocytes in atherosclerotic plaques express higher levels of CX3CR1 and CX3CL1 promoting chemotaxis of monocytes and T-lymphocytes to the plaque [72].CX3CL1 can be expressed by epithelial cells, but vascular endothelial cells and smooth muscle cells do not normally express CX3CL1. TNFα can induce expression of CX3CR1/L1 in these tissues [70], which corresponds with detection of CX3CR1/L1 at a later stage of plaque formation. Sacre *et al.* reported that $CD4^+CX3CR1^+$T-cells produced more TNFα and IFN γ *in vitro* than $CD4^+CX3CR1^-$ T-cells. This is consistent with a potential feedback mechanism in which $CD4^+CX3CR1^+$ T-cells exacerbate plaque formation. Immuno-histochemical staining of coronary arterial wall samples from HIV patients with atherosclerosis showed a presence of CX3CR1, CD4 and CD3 at *early* stages of atherogenesis, so $CD4^+CX3CR1^+$ T-cells could initiate plaque formation [73].

4. HIV patients stable on ART have a stronger footprint of CMV

In HIV patients with suppressed HIV replication on ART, the recovery of $CD4^+$ T-cell counts is limited by replenishment from the thymus and the loss of T-cells through persistent chronic immune activation [74, 75].Persistent CD4+ T-cell deficiency is most common in patients with low nadir CD4+ T-cell counts (<100 cells/µl) even though some patients beginning ART with severe T-cell depletion achieve effective immune reconstitution [76]. Patients with abundant thymic tissue show a faster and higher return of naïve $CD4^+$ T-cells after ART. However the thymus is a site of HIV replication. Infected thymocytes may die (through necrosis or apoptosis) or survive and carry the HIV provirus to their progenies (establishing latent infection). As HIV disease progresses, the thymus becomes prematurely atrophic, with changes similar to those seen in old age. For example, the thymus of a 30 year-old with late stage AIDS may be morphologically similar to the normal atrophic thymus of a 60 year-old [77].

Thymic dysfunction and the consequent release of autoreactive T-cells into circulation are implicated in the autoimmune and immunopathological conditions normally seen in old age - conditions that are more common in HIV patients (including those with a virological response to ART) than in the general population. This includes cardiovascular disease – which is influenced by the ART regime, life-style factors (smoking, exercise etc.) and other infections, notably CMV. CMV infection is more prominent in HIV patients, so its role in immunological aging and cardiovascular disease requires evaluation [78].

Over 50% of healthy individuals and 90% of individuals living with HIV are seropositive for CMV. Retinitis is the most common manifestation of CMV disease in HIV-infected individuals, affecting up to 40% of American AIDS patients, and many HIV patients in the developing world [3, 79].Treatment of systemic CMV disease is expensive and protracted, so prophylaxis is suspended once patients are stable on ART. As discussed earlier, CMV has the capacity for latency with frequent reactivation triggered by inflammatory mediators, including TNF [80]. Immune activation in treated and untreated HIV disease increases levels of this cytokine in circulation and tissues [81], so frequent subclinical reactivation of CMV is expected.

It appears likely that CMV and thymic insufficiency are synergistic in their effects on T-cell profiles in HIV patients. This is supported by evidence that homeostatic expansion of existing T-cells maintains T-cell numbers in the absence of thymic output, so age-related declines in immune function are accentuated in patients thymectomised in early childhood. This was clearest in individuals with strong T-cell responses to CMV IE and pp65 antigens [82].Accumulation of CMV –specific T-cells with an immunosenescent phenotype is greater in HIV patients than in age-matched controls [83, 84]. The importance of CMV in immune activation and immunosenesence in HIV patients is confirmed by evidence that immune activation was reduced when patients were treated with valgancyclovir [85].

Our studies of HIV patients also suggest that elevated T-cell and humoral responses to CMV reflect frequent reactivation. We investigated HIV patients who began antiretroviral therapy (ART) with extreme immunodeficiency and maintained a virological response until they were >50 years old. One can assume that they had a high burden of CMV pre-ART as many had experienced CMV retinitis. These HIV patients retained high titres of antibody reactive with CMV after 14 [13-16] years on ART and displayed elevated IFNγ responses to an immediate early peptide of CMV*(unpublished data)*.Such patients display accelerated cardiovascular disease that correlates with responses to CMV [86].

CD4+CX3CR1+ T-cells may help explain the role of CMV-specific cells in development of atherosclerosis in HIV patients, but the mechanisms requires further investigation. Interest in CX3CR/L in atherosclerosis is focussed by three findings reported in several studies.

1. Atherosclerosis is an inflammatory disease that is more frequent in HIV patients and cannot be attributed to ART cardiotoxicity alone [87, 88, 89, 90, 91].

2. HIV patients have a high proportion of CMV-specific T-cells [82, 83, 92]

3. CX3CR1 is found in atherosclerotic lesions and is expressed by T-cells [69,70]

A study of CX3CR1+ CD4+ T-cells and their implications in CVD was conducted in HIV-infected (n=29) and uninfected (n=48) individuals. The frequency of $CD4^{+}CX3CR1^{+}$ T-cells correlated with increasing carotid intima-media thickness (cIMT) in HIV-infected individuals.

These cells were antigen primed ($CD45RA^-$, $CD27^-$), activated (HLA-DR+) and immunosenescent ($CD57^+$) [73].

It may also be important that NK function is deficient in HIV patients. HIV infection changes the proportions of NK cell subsets, and expression of their activating and inhibitory receptors. It also perturbs their cytotoxic functions and cytokine production [93].Our group has published two studies of previously immunodeficient Australian patients, stabilised for many years on ART:

1. CD4+ T-cell IFNγ responses to CMV were *inversely* related to CD4+ T-cell counts before ART in patients who began ART with <60 CD4+ T-cells/μL, but IFNγ responses of NK cells to an unrestricted target (K562 cells) were *directly* proportional to nadir CD4+ T-cell counts [94].This establishes that NK cells don't follow the same trends as CD4+ T-cells on ART and do keep the imprint of the pre-ART immune system for many years.

2. NK cell IFNγ responses and proportions of $CD56^{lo}CD16^+$ NK cells were positively correlated and lower in patients than controls (confirming persistent NK dysfunction). Proportions of $CD56^{hi}CD16^{neg}$ NK cells (a phenotype associated with cytokine production) correlated inversely with CD4+ T-cell counts after ART and expression of perforin in this NK subset was *higher* in HIV patients than healthy controls. So these NK cells may compensate for T-cell deficiency [95].

5. CMV remains an important pathogen after renal transplantation

CMV reactivation (in previously seropositive recipients) or primary infection (in any recipient) is the most common infectious complication in renal transplantation [96].In the 1970's one in three recipients experienced pathologies associated with CMV. In one study of 141 patients, 12 *died* with disseminated CMV infection [97, 98].

In Australia, prophylaxis (valganciclovir) is routinely administered for 12-26 weeks after transplantation, according to a formula that considers donor and recipient CMV seropositivity and clinical risk. Under an equivalent regime, CMV recurred in 14/43 (33%) seropositive patients and in 4/19 (21%) patients after primary infection [99]. CMV remains a significant cause of graft loss despite prophylaxis and in the longer term, CMV reactivations are implicated in deterioration in renal function [100, 101], exhaustion or senescence of T-cells and cardiovascular disease.

Cardiovascular disease is recognised as a long term complication of renal transplantation, but a recent review [102] attributed this to immunosuppression. CMV antigenaemia (pp65) in the first year post-transplant did not predict cardiovascular disease over the next 2 years [102], but the study did no assess the longer term footprint of CMV disease. It is notable that Gomez et al [103] associated cardiovascular disease with CMV seropositivity over 1 year post-transplant in patients given oral ganciclovir.

http://dx.doi.org/10.5772/54798

6. Conclusions

The immune response to CMV has been studied extensively in mice and evidence is now accumulating from studies in humans. It is clear that NK cell and T cell responses are both important and that they influence each other. We propose a "footprint of CMV" as a tool to investigate the short and long term effects of CMV infection.

The footprint may include

1. CMV DNA detected by a sensitive PCR assay of blood, saliva or urine.
2. CMV-peptide/HLA tetramer positive CD8 T cells: The number of these cells in the blood is thought to reflect an accumulation of cells responding to CMV replication.
3. IFN-γ responses of $CD4^+$ and $CD8^+$ T-cells to CMV antigens enumerated by ELISPOT or flow cytometry.
4. Anti-CMV antibody detected by ELISA
5. Expression of NKG2C and LIR-1 on NK cells and T cells: NKG2C is expressed on a very small proportion of NK cells in CMV-seronegative subjects but expressed on a substantial proportion of NK cells from CMV seropositive subjects [31,32,33]and is considered a hallmark of CMV exposure. This probably reflects expansion of a small NK cell population in response to CMV infection. LIR-1 expression is also increased in subjects with higher titres of CMV antibody.

The resulting holistic view of the immune response in man will be a foundation for future studies aimed at identifying phenotypes associated with protection and those individuals who will benefit most from CMV prophylaxis.

Author details

Patricia Price

University of Western Australia, Australia

References

[1] Murphy E, Yu D, Grimwood J, Schmutz J, Dickson M, Jarvis MA, Hahn G, Nelson JA, Myers RM, Shenk TE. Coding potential of laboratory and clinical strains of human cytomegalovirus. Proc Natl Acad Sci USA, 2003; 100 14976-81.

[2] Landolfo S, Gariglio M, Gribaudo G, Lembo D. The human cytomegalovirus. Pharmacol Therap 2003; 269-297

[3] Ganekal S, Jhanji V, Dorairaj S, Nagarajappa A. Evaluation of Ocular Manifestations and Blindness in HIV/AIDS Patients in a Tertiary Care Hospital in South India. Ocul Immunol Inflamm. 2012; 1-6

[4] Price P, Olver SD. Animal Models for Human Immunopathological diseases: Cytomegalovirus Disease. ClinImmunolImmunopath 1996; 80:215-24.

[5] Scalzo AA, Yokoyama WM. Cmv1 and natural killer cell responses to murine cytomegalovirusinfection.Curr Top Microbiol Immunol 2008; 321:101-22

[6] Farrell HE, Abraham AM, Cardin RD, Sparre-Ulrich AH, Rosenkilde MM, Spiess K, Jensen TH, Kledal TN, Davis-Poynter N. Partial functional complementation between human and mouse cytomegalovirus chemokine receptor homologues. J Virol. 2011; 85(12): 6091-6095

[7] Price P. Are MHC proteins cellular receptors for CMV? Immunol Today. 1994; 15(6): 295-6.

[8] Van Bruggen I, Price P, Robertson TA, Papadimitriou JM. Morphological and functional changes during cytomegalovirus replication in murine macrophages. J Leukoc Biol. 1989; 46:508-20.

[9] Andrews DM, Andoniou CE, Granucci F, Ricciardi-Castagnoli P, Degli-Esposti MA. Infection of dendritic cells by murine cytomegalovirus induces functional paralysis. Nat Immunol. 2001; 2(11):1077-84.

[10] Price P, Baxter AG, Allcock RN, Papadimitriou JM. Factors influencing the effects of murine cytomegalovirus on the pancreas. Eur J Clin Invest. 1998 ;28:546-53.

[11] Price P, Olver SD, Silich M, Nador TZ, Yerkovich S, Wilson SG. Adrenalitis and the adrenocortical response of resistant and susceptible mice to acute murine cytomegalovirus infection. Eur J Clin Invest. 1996;26:811-19

[12] Gamadia LE, Rentenaar RJ, Baars PA, Remmerswaal EBM, Surachno S, Weel JF, Toebes M, Differentiation of cytomegalovirus-specific CD8+ T cells in healthy and immunosuppressed virus carriers. Blood. 2001;98(3):754-61.

[13] Lin A, Xu H, Yan W. Modulation of HLA expression in human cytomegalovirus immune evasion. Cell Mol Immunol. 2007;4(2):91-8.

[14] Gamadia LE, Remmerswaal EB, Weel JF, Bemelman F, van Lier RA, Ten Berge IJ. Primary immune responses to human CMV: a critical role for IFN-gamma-producing CD4+ T cells in protection against CMV disease. Blood. 2003;101(7):2686-92

[15] Sumaria N, van Dommelen SL, Andoniou CE, Smyth MJ, Scalzo AA, Degli-Esposti MA. The roles of interferon-gamma and perforin in antiviral immunity in mice that differ in genetically determined NK-cell-mediated antiviral activity. Immunol Cell Biol. 2009; 87(7):559-66.

[16] Pyzik M, Gendron-Pontbriand EM, Vidal SM. The impact of Ly49-NK cell-dependent recognition of MCMV infection on innate and adaptive immune responses. J Biomed Biotechnol. 2011;2011:641702.

[17] Arens R, Loewendorf A, Her MJ, Schneider-Ohrum K, Shellam GR, Janssen E, Ware CF, Schoenberger SP, Benedict CA. B7-mediated costimulation of CD4 T cells constrains cytomegalovirus persistence. J Virol. 2011;85(1):390-6.

[18] Lemmermann NA, Böhm V, Holtappels R, Reddehase MJ. In vivo impact of cytomegalovirus evasion of CD8 T-cell immunity: facts and thoughts based on murine models. Virus Res. 2011;157(2):161-74.

[19] Kuijpers TW, Baars PA, Dantin C, van den Burg M, van Lier RA, Roosnek E. Human NK cells can control CMV infection in the absence of T cells. Blood. 2008 Aug 1;112(3): 914-5.

[20] Revilleza MJ, Wang R, Mans J, Hong M, Natarajan K, Margulies DH. How the virus outsmarts the host: function and structure of cytomegalovirus MHC-I-like molecules in the evasion of natural killer cell surveillance. J Biomed Biotechnol. 2011;2011:724607

[21] Wilkinson GW, Tomasec P, Stanton RJ, Armstrong M, Prod'homme V, Aicheler R, McSharry BP, Rickards CR, Cochrane D, Llewellyn-Lacey S, Wang EC, Griffin CA, Davison AJ. Modulation of natural killer cells by human cytomegalovirus. J Clin Virol. 2008 Mar;41(3):206-12.

[22] Affandi JS, Aghafar ZK, Rodriguez B, Lederman MM, Burrows S, Senitzer D, Price P. Can immune-related genotypes illuminate the immunopathogenesis of cytomegalovirus disease in human immunodeficiency virus-infected patients? Hum Immunol. 2012 Feb; 73(2):168-74.

[23] Stern M, Elsässer H, Hönger G, Steiger J, Schaub S, Hess C. The number of activating KIR genes inversely correlates with the rate of CMV infection/reactivation in kidney transplant recipients. Am J Transplant. 2008 Jun;8(6):1312-7.

[24] Zaia JA, Sun JY, Gallez-Hawkins GM, Thao L, Oki A, Lacey SF, Dagis A, Palmer J, Diamond DJ, Forman SJ, Senitzer D. The effect of single and combined activating killer immunoglobulin-like receptor genotypes on cytomegalovirus infection and immunity after hematopoietic cell transplantation. Biol Blood Marrow Transplant. 2009 Mar;15(3): 315-25.

[25] Cook M, Briggs D, Craddock C, Mahendra P, Milligan D, Fegan C, Darbyshire P, Lawson S, Boxall E, Moss P. Donor KIR genotype has a major influence on the rate of cytomegalovirus reactivation following T-cell replete stem cell transplantation. Blood. 2006 Feb 1;107(3):1230-2.

[26] Chen C, Busson M, Rocha V, Appert ML, Lepage V, Dulphy N, Haas P, Socié G, Toubert A, Charron D, Loiseau P. Activating KIR genes are associated with CMV reactivation and survival after non-T-cell depleted HLA-identical sibling bone marrow transplantation for malignant disorders. Bone Marrow Transplant. 2006 Sep;38(6):437-44.

[27] Jamil KM, Khakoo SI. KIR/HLA interactions and pathogen immunity. J Biomed Biotechnol. 2011; 298348.

[28] Foley B, De Santis D, Lathbury L, Christiansen F, Witt C. KIR2DS1-mediated activation overrides NKG2A-mediated inhibition in HLA-C C2-negative individuals. Int Immunol. 2008 Apr;20(4):555-63.

[29] Chewning JH, Gudme CN, Hsu KC, Selvakumar A, Dupont B. KIR2DS1-positive NK cells mediate alloresponse against the C2 HLA-KIR ligand group in vitro. J Immunol. 2007 Jul 15;179(2):854-68.

[30] Prod'homme V, Griffin C, Aicheler RJ, Wang EC, McSharry BP, Rickards CR, Stanton RJ, Borysiewicz LK, López-Botet M, Wilkinson GW, Tomasec P. The human cytomegalovirus MHC class I homolog UL18 inhibits LIR-1+ but activates LIR-1- NK cells. J Immunol. 2007 Apr 1;178(7):4473-81.

[31] Wagner CS, Riise GC, Bergström T, Kärre K, Carbone E, Berg L. Increased expression of leukocyte Ig-like receptor-1 and activating role of UL18 in the response to cytomegalovirus infection. J Immunol. 2007 Mar 15;178(6):3536-43.

[32] Berg L, Riise GC, Cosman D, Bergström T, Olofsson S, Kärre K, Carbone E. LIR-1 expression on lymphocytes, and cytomegalovirus disease in lung-transplant recipients. Lancet. 2003 Mar 29;361(9363):1099-101.

[33] Gumá M, Budt M, Sáez A, Brckalo T, Hengel H, Angulo A, López-Botet M. Expansion of CD94/NKG2C+ NK cells in response to human cytomegalovirus-infected fibroblasts. Blood. 2006 May 1;107(9):3624-31.

[34] Hadaya K, de Rham C, Bandelier C, Bandelier C, Ferrari-Lacraz S, Jendly S, Berney T, Buhler L, Kaiser L, Seebach JD, Tiercy JM, Martin PY, Villard J.Natural killer cell receptor repertoire and their ligands, and the risk of CMV infection after kidney transplantation. Am J Transplant. 2008 Dec;8(12):2674-83.

[35] Adam E, Melnick JL, Probtsfield JL, Petrie BL, Burek J, Bailey KR, McCollum CH, DeBakey ME. High levels of cytomegalovirus antibody in patients requiring vascular surgery for atherosclerosis. Lancet. 1987 Aug 8; 2(8554):291-3.

[36] Price P, Eddy KS, Papadimitriou JM, Faulkner DL, Shellam GR. Genetic determination of cytomegalovirus-induced and age-related cardiopathy in inbred mice. Characterization of infiltrating cells. Am J Pathol. 1991 Jan; 138(1):59-67.

[37] Ross R. Atherosclerosis--an inflammatory disease. N Engl J Med. 1999 Jan 14; 340(2): 115-26.

[38] Libby P. Inflammation in atherosclerosis. Arterioscler Thromb Vasc Biol. 2012 Sep; 32(9):2045-51.

[39] Liu H, Jiang D. Fractalkine/CX3CR1 and atherosclerosis. Clin Chim Acta. 2011 Jun 11;412(13-14):1180-6.

[40] Kraemer, R. Regulation of Cell Migration in Atherosclerosis Current Atherosclerosis Reports 2000 2(5):445–452

[41] Schindhelm RK, van der Zwan LP, Teerlink T, Scheffer PG. Myeloperoxidase: a useful biomarker for cardiovascular disease risk stratification? Clin Chem. 2009 Aug;55(8): 1462-70.

[42] Meng L, Park J, Cai Q, Lanting L, Reddy MA, Natarajan R. Diabetic conditions promote binding of monocytes to vascular smooth muscle cells and their subsequent differentiation. Am J Physiol Heart Circ Physiol. 2010 Mar; 298(3):H736-45.

[43] Maggi P, Perilli F, Lillo A, Carito V, Epifani G, Bellacosa C, Pastore G, Regina G. An ultrasound-based comparative study on carotid plaques in HIV-positive patients vs. atherosclerotic and arteritis patients: atherosclerotic or inflammatory lesions? Coron Artery Dis. 2007 Feb;18(1):23-9.

[44] Toyoda M, Galfayan K, Galera OA, Petrosian A, Czer LS, Jordan SC. Cytomegalovirus infection induces anti-endothelial cell antibodies in cardiac and renal allograft recipients. Transpl Immunol. 1997 Jun;5(2):104-11

[45] Varani S, Muratori L, De Ruvo N, Vivarelli M, Lazzarotto T, Gabrielli L, Bianchi FB, Bellusci R, Landini MP. Autoantibody appearance in cytomegalovirus-infected liver transplant recipients: correlation with antigenemia. J Med Virol. 2002 Jan; 66(1):56-62.

[46] Varani S, Landini MP. Cytomegalovirus-induced immunopathology and its clinical consequences. Herpesviridae. 2011 Apr 7;2(1):6

[47] Simantov R, Lo SK, Gharavi A, Sammaritano LR, Salmon JE, Silverstein RL. Antiphospholipid antibodies activate vascular endothelial cells. Lupus. 1996 Oct;5(5):440-1.

[48] Olsson J, Wikby A, Johansson B, Löfgren S, Nilsson BO, Ferguson FG. Age-related change in peripheral blood T-lymphocyte subpopulations and cytomegalovirus infection in the very old: the Swedish longitudinal OCTO immune study. Mech Ageing Dev. 2000 Dec 20;121(1-3):187-201.

[49] Pawelec G, McElhaney JE, Aiello AE, Derhovanessian E. The impact of CMV infection on survival in older humans. Curr Opin Immunol. 2012 Aug;24(4):507-11.

[50] Hadrup SR, Strindhall J, Køllgaard T, Seremet T, Johansson B, Pawelec G, thor Straten P, Wikby A. Longitudinal studies of clonally expanded CD8 T cells reveal a repertoire shrinkage predicting mortality and an increased number of dysfunctional cytomegalovirus-specific T cells in the very elderly. J Immunol. 2006 Feb 15;176(4):2645-53.

[51] Roberts ET, Haan MN, Dowd JB, Aiello AE. Cytomegalovirus antibody levels, inflammation, and mortality among elderly Latinos over 9 years of follow-up. Am J Epidemiol. 2010 Aug 15;172(4):363-71.

[52] Berry NJ, Burns DM, Wannamethee G, Grundy JE, Lui SF, Prentice HG, Griffiths PD. Seroepidemiologic studies on the acquisition of antibodies to cytomegalovirus, herpes simplex virus, and human immunodeficiency virus among general hospital patients

and those attending a clinic for sexually transmitted diseases. J Med Virol. 1988 Apr; 24(4):385-93.

[53] Moro-García MA, Alonso-Arias R, López-Vázquez A, Suárez-García FM, Solano-Jaurrieta JJ, Baltar J, López-Larrea C. Relationship between functional ability in older people, immune system status, and intensity of response to CMV. Age (Dordr). 2012 Apr;34(2):479-95.

[54] Khan N, Shariff N, Cobbold M, Bruton R, Ainsworth JA, Sinclair AJ, Nayak L, Moss PA. Cytomegalovirus seropositivity drives the CD8 T cell repertoire toward greater clonality in healthy elderly individuals. J Immunol. 2002 Aug 15;169(4):1984-92.

[55] Vescovini R, Biasini C, Telera AR, Basaglia M, Stella A, Magalini F, Bucci L, Monti D, Lazzarotto T, Dal Monte P, Pedrazzoni M, Medici MC, Chezzi C, Franceschi C, Fagnoni FF, Sansoni P. Intense antiextracellular adaptive immune response to human cytomegalovirus in very old subjects with impaired health and cognitive and functional status. J Immunol. 2010 Mar 15;184(6):3242-9.

[56] Ouyang Q, Wagner WM, Zheng W, Wikby A, Remarque EJ, Pawelec G. Dysfunctional CMV-specific CD8(+) T cells accumulate in the elderly. Exp Gerontol. 2004 Apr;39(4): 607-13.

[57] Pawelec G, Derhovanessian E. Role of CMV in immune senescence. Virus Res, 2011,157(2):175–9

[58] Ouyang Q, Wagner WM, Zheng W, Wikby A, Remarque EJ, Pawelec G. Dysfunctional CMV-specific CD8(+) T cells accumulate in the elderly. Exp Gerontol. 2004 Apr;39(4): 607-13.

[59] Jarvis MA, Nelson JA. Human cytomegalovirus tropism for endothelial cells: not all endothelial cells are created equal. J Virol. 2007 Mar;81(5):2095-101.

[60] eckert CK, Renzaho A, Tervo HM, Krause C, Deegen P, Kühnapfel B, Reddehase MJ, Grzimek NK. Liver sinusoidal endothelial cells are a site of murine cytomegalovirus latency and reactivation. J Virol. 2009 Sep;83(17):8869-84.

[61] Koffron AJ, Hummel M, Patterson BK, Yan S, Kaufman DB, Fryer JP, Stuart FP, Abecassis MI. Cellular localization of latent murine cytomegalovirus. J Virol. 1998 Jan; 72(1):95-103.

[62] Gyorkey F, Melnick JL, Guinn GA, Gyorkey P, DeBakey ME. Herpesviridae in the endothelial and smooth muscle cells of the proximal aorta in arteriosclerotic patients. Exp Mol Pathol. 1984 Jun;40(3):328-39.

[63] Hendrix MG, Dormans PH, Kitslaar P, Bosman F, Bruggeman CA. The presence of cytomegalovirus nucleic acids in arterial walls of atherosclerotic and nonatherosclerotic patients. Am J Pathol. 1989 May;134(5):1151-7.

[64] Gredmark-Russ S, Dzabic M, Rahbar A, Wanhainen A, Björck M, Larsson E, Michel JB, Söderberg-Nauclér C. Active cytomegalovirus infection in aortic smooth muscle cells from patients with abdominal aortic aneurysm. J Mol Med (Berl). 2009 Apr;87(4):347-56.

[65] Haarala A, Kähönen M, Lehtimäki T, Aittoniemi J, Jylhävä J, Hutri-Kähönen N, Taittonen L, Laitinen T, Juonala M, Viikari J, Raitakari OT, Hurme M. Relation of high cytomegalovirus antibody titres to blood pressure and brachial artery flow-mediated dilation in young men: the Cardiovascular Risk in Young Finns Study. Clin Exp Immunol. 2012 Feb;167(2):309-16.

[66] Safaie N, Ghotaslou R, Montazer Ghaem H. Seroprevalence of cytomegalovirus in patients with and without coronary artery diseases at Madani Heart Center, Iran. Acta Med Iran. 2010 Nov-Dec;48(6):403-6.

[67] Romo N, Fitó M, Gumá M, Sala J, García C, Ramos R, Muntasell A, Masiá R, Bruguera J, Subirana I, Vila J, de Groot E, Elosua R, Marrugat J, López-Botet M. Association of atherosclerosis with expression of the LILRB1 receptor by human NK and T-cells supports the infectious burden hypothesis. Arterioscler Thromb Vasc Biol. 2011 Oct; 31(10):2314-21.

[68] Hsue PY, Hunt PW, Sinclair E, Bredt B, Franklin A, Killian M, Hoh R, Martin JN, McCune JM, Waters DD, Deeks SG. Increased carotid intima-media thickness in HIV patients is associated with increased cytomegalovirus-specific T-cell responses. AIDS. 2006 Nov 28;20(18):2275-83.

[69] Wong BW, Wong D, McManus BM. Characterization of fractalkine (CX3CL1) and CX3CR1 in human coronary arteries with native atherosclerosis, diabetes mellitus, and transplant vascular disease. Cardiovasc Pathol. 2002 Nov-Dec;11(6):332-8.

[70] Ludwig A, Berkhout T, Moores K, Groot P, Chapman G. Fractalkine is expressed by smooth muscle cells in response to IFN-gamma and TNF-alpha and is modulated by metalloproteinase activity. J Immunol. 2002 Jan 15;168(2):604-12.

[71] olovan-Fritts CA, Spector SA. Endothelial damage from cytomegalovirus-specific host immune response can be prevented by targeted disruption of fractalkine-CX3CR1 interaction. Blood. 2008 Jan 1;111(1):175-82.

[72] ostolakis S, Krambovitis E, Vlata Z, Kochiadakis GE, Baritaki S, Spandidos DA. CX3CR1 receptor is up-regulated in monocytes of coronary artery diseased patients: impact of pre-inflammatory stimuli and renin-angiotensin system modulators. Thromb Res. 2007;121(3):387-95.

[73] Sacre K, Hunt PW, Hsue PY, Maidji E, Martin JN, Deeks SG, Autran B, McCune JM. A role for cytomegalovirus-specific CD4+CX3CR1+ T cells and cytomegalovirus-induced T-cell immunopathology in HIV-associated atherosclerosis. AIDS. 2012 Apr 24;26(7): 805-14.

[74] Gordon SN, Cervasi B, Odorizzi P, Silverman R, Aberra F, Ginsberg G, Estes JD, Paiardini M, Frank I, Silvestri G. Disruption of intestinal CD4+ T cell homeostasis is a

key marker of systemic CD4+ T cell activation in HIV-infected individuals. J Immunol 2010; 185:5169-79

[75] Fernandez S, Nolan RC, Price P, Krueger R, Wood C, Cameron D, Solomon A, Lewin SR and French MA. Thymic function in severely immunodeficient HIV type 1-infected patients receiving stable and effective antiretroviral therapy. AIDS Res Hum Retroviruses 2006; 22:163-70

[76] Kaufmann GR, Furrer H, Ledergerber B, Perrin L, Opravil M, Vernazza P, Cavassini M, Bernasconi E, Rickenbach M, Hirschel B and Battegay M. Characteristics, determinants, and clinical relevance of CD4 T cell recovery to <500 cells/microL in HIV type 1-infected individuals receiving potent antiretroviral therapy. Clin Infect Dis 2005; 41:361-72.

[77] Meissner EG, Duus KM, Loomis R, D'Agostin R and Su L. HIV-1 replication and pathogenesis in the human thymus. Curr HIV Res 2003; 1:275-85.

[78] Haynes BF, Markert ML, Sempowski GD, Patel DD and Hale LP. The role of the thymus in immune reconstitution in aging, bone marrow transplantation, and HIV-1 infection. Annu Rev Immunol 2000; 18:529-60.

[79] Heiden D, Ford N, Wilson D, Rodriguez WR, Margolis T, Janssens B, Bedelu M, Tun N, Goemaere E, Saranchuk P, Sabapathy K, Smithuis F, Luyirika E and Drew WL. Cytomegalovirus retinitis: the neglected disease of the AIDS pandemic. PLoS Med 2007; 4:e334

[80] Docke WD, Prosch S, Fietze E, Kimel V, Zuckermann H, Klug C, Syrbe U, Kruger DH, von Baehr R and Volk HD. Cytomegalovirus reactivation and tumour necrosis factor. Lancet 1994; 343:268-9.

[81] Ownby RL, Kumar AM, Benny Fernandez J, Moleon-Borodowsky I, Gonzalez L, Eisdorfer S, Waldrop-Valverde D and Kumar M. Tumor necrosis factor-alpha levels in HIV-1 seropositive injecting drug users. J NeuroimmunePharmacol 2009; 4:350-8.

[82] Sauce D, Larsen M, Fastenackels S, Duperrier A, Keller M, Grubeck-Loebenstein B, Ferrand C, Debre P, Sidi D and Appay V. Evidence of premature immune aging in patients thymectomized during early childhood. J Clin Invest 2009; 119:3070-8.

[83] Stone SF, Price P and French MA. Cytomegalovirus (CMV)-specific CD8+ T cells in individuals with HIV infection: correlation with protection from CMV disease. J Anti microb Chemother 2006; 57:585-8.

[84] Naeger DM, Martin JN, Sinclair E, Hunt PW, Bangsberg DR, Hecht F, Hsue P, McCune JM, Deeks SG. Cytomegalovirus-specific T cells persist at very high levels during long-term antiretroviral treatment of HIV disease. PLoS One. 2010 Jan 29;5(1):e8886.

[85] Hunt PW, Martin JN, Sinclair E, Epling L, Teague J, Jacobson MA, Tracy RP, Corey L, Deeks SG. Valganciclovir reduces T cell activation in HIV-infected individuals with incomplete CD4+ T cell recovery on antiretroviral therapy. J Infect Dis. 2011 May 15;203(10):1474-83.

[86] Hsue PY, Hunt PW, Sinclair E, Bredt B, Franklin A, Killian M, Hoh R, Martin JN, McCune JM, Waters DD and Deeks SG. Increased carotid intima-media thickness in HIV patients is associated with increased cytomegalovirus-specific T-cell responses. AIDS 2006; 20:2275-83.

[87] Parrinello CM, Sinclair E, Landay AL, Lurain N, Sharrett AR, Gange SJ, Xue X, Hunt PW, Deeks SG, Hodis HN, Kaplan RC. Cytomegalovirus immunoglobulin G antibody is associated with subclinical carotid artery disease among HIV-infected women. J Infect Dis. 2012 Jun 15;205(12):1788-96.

[88] Triant VA, Lee H, Hadigan C, Grinspoon SK. Increased acute myocardial infarction rates and cardiovascular risk factors among patients with human immunodeficiency virus disease. J Clin Endocrinol Metab. 2007 Jul;92(7):2506-12.

[89] Fisher SD, Miller TL, Lipshultz SE. Impact of HIV and highly active antiretroviral therapy on leukocyte adhesion molecules, arterial inflammation, dyslipidemia, and atherosclerosis. Atherosclerosis. 2006 Mar;185(1):1-11.

[90] Vittecoq D, Escaut L, Chironi G, Teicher E, Monsuez JJ, Andrejak M, Simon A. Coronary heart disease in HIV-infected patients in the highly active antiretroviral treatment era. AIDS. 2003 Apr;17 Suppl 1:S70-6.

[91] Zona S, Raggi P, Bagni P, Orlando G, Carli F, Ligabue G, Scaglioni R, Rossi R, Modena MG, Guaraldi G. Parallel increase of subclinical atherosclerosis and epicardial adipose tissue in patients with HIV. Am Heart J. 2012 Jun;163(6):1024-30.

[92] Tan DB, Fernandez S, French M and Price P. Could natural killer cells compensate for impaired CD4+ T-cell responses to CMV in HIV patients responding to antiretroviral therapy? ClinImmunol 2009; 132:63-70.

[93] Fauci AS, Mavilio D and Kottilil S. NK cells in HIV infection: paradigm for protection or targets for ambush. Nat Rev Immunol 2005; 5:835-43.

[94] Price P, Fernandez S, Tan DB, James IR, Keane NM and French MA. Nadir CD4 T-cell counts continue to influence interferon-gamma responses in HIV patients who began antiretroviral treatment with advanced immunodeficiency. J Acquir Immune Defic-Syndr 2008; 49:462-4.

[95] Tan DB, Fernandez S, French M and Price P. Could natural killer cells compensate for impaired CD4+ T-cell responses to CMV in HIV patients responding to antiretroviral therapy? ClinImmunol 2009; 132:63-70.

[96] Fishman JA. Infection in solid-organ transplant recipients. N Eng J Med 2007; 357:2601-14

[97] Peterson PK, Balfour HH Jr, Marker SC, Fryd DS, Howard RJ, Simmons RL. Cytomegalovirus disease in renal allograft recipients: a prospective study of the clinical features, risk factors and impact on renal transplantation. Medicine (Baltimore). 1980 Jul;59(4):283-300.

[98] Helanterä I, Lautenschlager I, Koskinen P. The risk of cytomegalovirus recurrence after kidney transplantation. Transpl Int. 2011 Dec;24(12):1170-8.

[99] Luan FL, Kommareddi M, Ojo AO. Impact of cytomegalovirus disease in D+/R- kidney transplant patients receiving 6 months low-dose valganciclovir prophylaxis. Am J Transplant. 2011 Sep;11(9):1936-42.

[100] Smith JM, Corey L, Bittner R, Finn LS, Healey PJ, Davis CL, McDonald RA. Subclinical viremia increases risk for chronic allograft injury in pediatric renal transplantation. J Am Soc Nephrol. 2010 Sep;21(9):1579-86.

[101] Tong CY, Bakran A, Peiris JS, Muir P, Herrington CS. The association of viral infection and chronic allograft nephropathy with graft dysfunction after renal transplantation. Transplantation. 2002 Aug 27;74(4):576-8.

[102] Jardine AG, Gaston RS, Fellstrom BC, Holdaas H. Prevention of cardiovascular disease in adult recipients of kidney transplants. Lancet. 2011 Oct 15;378(9800):1419-27.

[103] Gómez E, Laurés A, Baltar JM, Melón S, Díez B, de Oña M. Cytomegalovirus replication and "herpesvirus burden" as risk factor of cardiovascular events in the first year after renal transplantation. Transplant Proc. 2005 Nov;37(9):3760-3.

Chapter 6

The Oncogenicity of Human Cytomegalovirus

Prakash Vishnu and David M. Aboulafia

Additional information is available at the end of the chapter

http://dx.doi.org/10.5772/55051

1. Introduction

The potential role of Human cytomegalovirus (hCM) infection in promoting neoplasia is an active area of scientific research. [1] Although still controversial, there is a growing body of evidence that links hCMV infection to a variety of malignancies, including those of the breast, prostate, colon, lung and brain (gliomas). [2-7] hCMV induces alterations in regulatory proteins and non-coding RNA that are associated with a malignant phenotype. These changes promote tumour survival by effecting cellular proliferation, invasion, immune evasion, and production of angiogenic factors [8] Constant immune surveillance governs the destruction of the majority of cancer cells and precancerous conditions in the human body. However, the most pathogenic of malignant tumors acquire immune evasion strategies which render them less vulnerable to destruction by immune cells.

The characteristic hallmarks of a malignant cell include:

1. sustaining proliferative signaling and evading growth suppressors,
2. resisting cell death and enabling replicative immortality,
3. inducing angiogenesis, activating invasion and metastasis. [9]

In cancers which are not attributable to infectious agents, chronic inflammation may also play a critical role in the transition from a precancerous condition to invasive malignancy. Inflammation is the seventh hallmark of neoplasia (Table 1). [10] During chronic inflammation, certain "promoters," such as hepatitis C virus and Epstein-Barr virus (EBV), may facilitate the transformation of a pre-malignant condition to neoplasia. [11,12] Cancer "promoters" are agents that, by themselves, may not have a significant oncogenic impact on normal cells but can drive precancerous cells towards neoplasia.

1. Sustaining proliferative signaling
2. Evading growth suppressors
3. Resisting cell death
4. Inducing angiogenesis
5. Activating invasion and metastasis
6. Enabling replicative immortality
7. Tumor-promoting inflammation

Table 1. The "seven" hallmarks of cancer

2. Chronic inflammation and oncogenesis

Associations linking chronic infection, chronic inflammation and malignancy have been well chronicled. [13] As many as 25% of all cancers can be traced to chronic infection or other types of chronic inflammation. [14] Infectious agents that cause chronic inflammation promote oncogenesis by complex pathways, and are depicted in Figure 1. Key mediators of inflammation-induced oncogenesis include generation of mutagenic chemical mediators such as reactive oxygen and nitrogen species, genetic variations in inflammatory cytokines [15], and creation of a micro-environment with features of chronic inflammation such as nuclear factor kappa B (NF-κB). [16,17] In such conditions, tumor-associated macrophages (TAMs) play a pivotal role in mediating inflammatory (M1) responses, as well as immunosuppressive and growth (M2) responses. [18]

M2-polarized TAMs and the related myeloid-derived suppressor cells are key components of smoldering inflammation that drives neoplastic progression. The M2 responses, while important for wound healing, can promote neoplastic transformation. TAMs respond to cytokines such as Interleukin (IL)-10 and Transforming Growth Factor (TGF)-β, acquiring M2 properties that promote immune suppression by blocking dendritic cell (DC) maturation and attracting regulatory T-cells (T-regs). [19,20] T-regs are potent inhibitors of the T-cell anti-tumor response. [21]

Activation of NF-κB pathway mediated by COX-2 and IL-6 via STAT-3 transcriptional activation also promotes malignant transformation. [22] NF-κB is a transcription factor that mediates an inflammatory cascade leading to generation of COX-2, an inducible isoform of nitric oxide synthase (iNOS) and the inflammatory cytokines IL-1β, IL-6, and Tumor Necrosis Factor (TNF) -α. These cytokines, in conjunction with nitric oxide produced by TAMs and tumor cells, are present in high concentration in the tumor microenvironment and are important promoters of inflammation-driven oncogenesis and immunosuppression. [23-25]

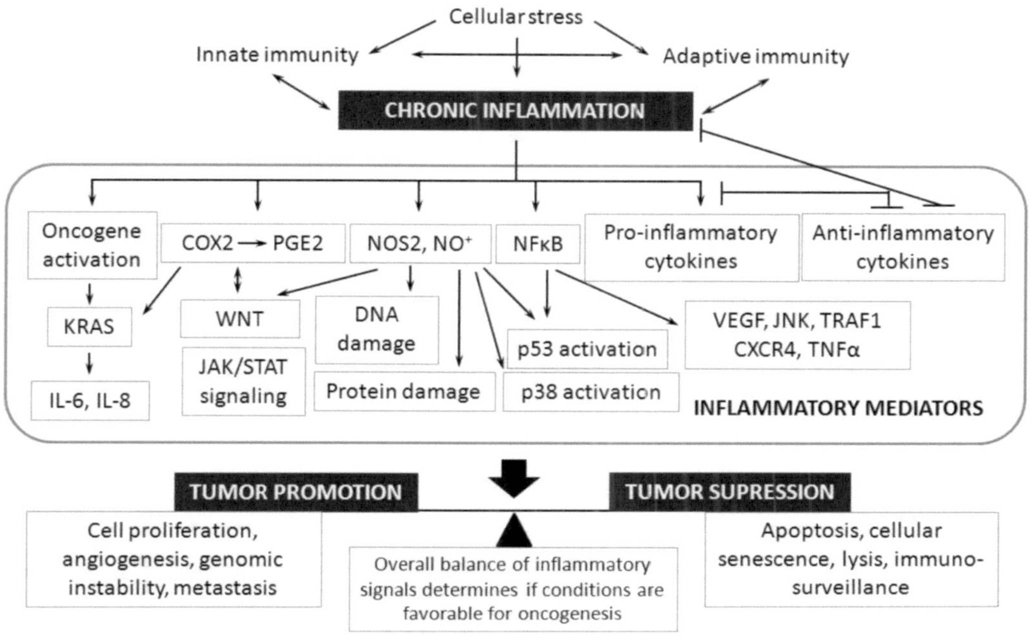

Figure 1. Pathway linking chronic inflammation and oncogenesis. (Adapted from Schetter et. al.[13])

3. Concept of oncomodulation

Tumor cells have aberrations in cell cycle signaling, RNA transcription and the production of tumor-suppression proteins. The concept of "oncomodulation" suggests that a virus may modulate cellular pathways [26] through changes to viral regulatory proteins and noncoding RNA which eludes to tumor cell properties (cell proliferation, survival, invasion, production of angiogenic factors, and immune evasion). hCMV not only promotes oncogenesis but also contributes to a more malignant tumor cell phenotype (Figure 2). While investigators have long postulated a role for hCMV in human neoplasia, many of the early studies were not reproducible and lacked clear *in situ* histopathological correlations with the proposed diseases. [27,28] The concept of "hit-and-run" oncogenesis holds that infection with hCMV takes place during an earlier time frame to tumour development. hCMV infection sets into motion processes resulting in malignancy, but the virus is no longer detectable by the time cancer occurs. [29] Several of the more important cellular pathways that could lead to cancer and which are modulated by hCMV are reviewed below.

3.1. Resistance to apoptosis

Resistance to apoptosis is a common feature of cancer cells. [9,30,31] Early research on hCMV infection revealed that hCMV protects the fibroblasts it infects from apoptosis. hCMV immediate early (IE) proteins (e.g., IE2-86 & IE2-72) [32] are able to prevent adenovirus E1A

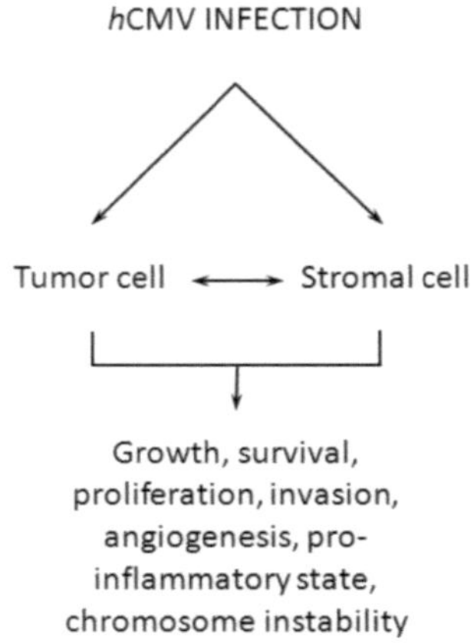

Figure 2. Concept of Oncomodulation. (Adapted from Michaelis et. al. [99])

protein-induced apoptosis-by both p53-dependent and independent mechanisms- of hCMV infected fibroblasts. Direct anti-apoptotic activity of hCMV proteins is related to defined transcripts encoded by the hCMV UL36-UL37 genes. [33,34] The product of the UL36 gene is an inhibitor of caspase activation which binds to the pro-domain of caspase-8 and inhibits Fas-mediated apoptosis. [35] Similarly, the UL37 gene product, UL37 exon 1, is a mitochondrial inhibitor of apoptosis and inhibits the recruitment of the pro-apoptotic proteins Bax and *Bak* to mitochondria, resulting in their functional inactivation. [36] hCMV further protects tumor cells from apoptosis by the induction of cellular proteins, including *AKT, Bcl-2, and* $\Delta Np73\alpha$. [37] Induction of the anti-apoptotic protein *Bcl-2* by hCMV, results in acquired resistance to cytotoxic drugs such as cisplatin and etoposide. This resistance can be reversed after treatment with the anti-hCMV drug, ganciclovir. [37] Engagement of platelet derived growth factor receptor (PDGFR) α or virus co-receptors (including integrins and Toll-like receptor-2) by hCMV glycoproteins can also lead to activation of mitogen-activated protein kinase (MAPK) and/or phosphatidyl-inositol 3-kinase (PI3-K) pathways that can alter apoptotic responses (Figure 3). [38-40]

3.2. Cancer cell adhesion, migration and invasion

Adhesion of cancer cells to endothelium is critical in promoting metastases. [41-43] hCMV can facilitate this process by promoting activation of integrins (e.g., $\beta 1\alpha 5$ and B1) on the tumor cell surface, and by increasing adhesion of tumor cells to the neighboring endothelium. Tumor cell adhesion to endothelium is also facilitated by activation of integrin-linked kinases (e.g., phosphorylation of focal adhesion kinase Tyr397). [4,,44] Down regulation of adhesion molecule receptors by hCMV (e.g., neural cell adhesion molecule, CD56), causes a focal disruption of endothelial cells facilitating tumor cell transmigration. [1,45] The net effects of hCMV on adhesion molecules account for decreased binding of cancer cells to each other and

http://dx.doi.org/10.5772/55051

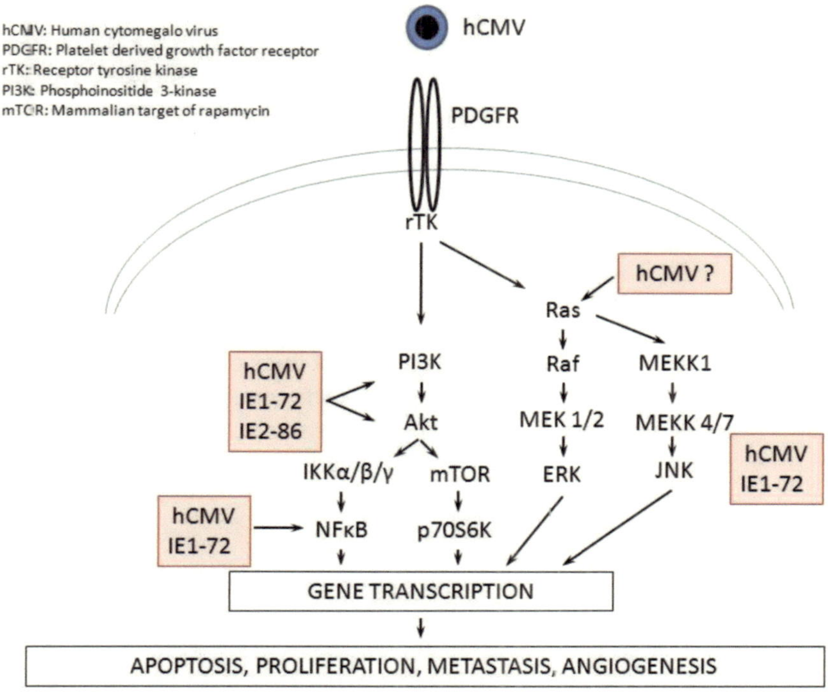

Figure 3. Major signaling pathways activated by hCMV that contribute to oncomodulation by hCMV. (Adapted from from Michaelis et. al [100])

increased binding to endothelium, which is an important early process in formation of metastasis.

3.3. Angiogenesis

Angiogenesis is the growth of the new blood vessels and is essential for growth of malignant tumors. [9,46] Through the technique of secretome analysis researchers have shown that proteins secreted from hCMV-infected cells contain increased levels of pro-angiogenic molecules, and increased pro-angiogenic activity in cell-free supernatants. [47] US28 is a hCMV protein seen in high concentrations in the supernatant. This particular protein alters adhesion properties of epithelial cells inducing a pro-angiogenic and transformed phenotype through up-regulation of vascular endothelial growth factor (VEGF). [48] Additional supernatant proteins, including IE1-72 and IE2-86, increase vascular smooth muscle cell migration, proliferation, and expression of PDGF-β receptor. Furthermore, IE2-86 promotes endothelial proliferation by binding and inactivating the tumor oncogene p53 in endothelial cells. [49,50] Expression of IL-8, another well-recognized promoter of tumor angiogenesis, is increased by hCMV via transactivation of IL-8 promoter through the cellular transcription factors NF-κB and AP-1. [51] Binding of hCMV to and signaling through integrin β1, integrin β3, and epidermal growth factor receptor can also promote angiogenesis. [47,52]

Expression of thrombospondin (TSP-1), a potent inhibitor of angiogenesis, is suppressed in several hCMV-infected cancer cell lines, suggesting yet another mechanism by which hCMV can promote increased angiogenesis and a more malignant phenotype. [53,54] hCMV - mediated activation of COX-2 may also promote angiogenesis in tumor cells by inducing expression of Fibroblast Growth Factor (FGF), VEGF, PDGF, iNOS, and TGF-α, and by promoting capillary endothelial cell migration and tube formation (Figure 3). [55]

3.4. Impact of hCMV on cell cycle

In hCMV-infected host cells, viral regulatory proteins induce cell cycle arrest and prevent cellular DNA replication, whilst replication of viral DNA remains enabled. [8,56] While some hCMV regulatory proteins can induce cell cycle arrest, others can promote cell cycle progression. [57,58] hCMV IE2-86 induces cell cycle arrest by activating ataxia telangiectasia mutated (ATM) gene-dependent phosphorylation of p53, leading to p53- and p21-dependent inhibition of cell cycle progression. [59] In contrast, the hCMV regulatory proteins IE1-72, IE2-86, and the tegument proteins *pp*71 and UL97 interact with and deactivate proteins of the Rb family, promoting entry into S-phase of the cell cycle. [60]

The cell cycle of neoplastic cells is inherently dysfunctional. [9,31] In precancerous or transformed cells, the function of virus regulatory proteins may depend on the replicative status of the cell. [61,62] The hCMV protein US28 promotes cell cycle progression and cyclin D1 expression in cells with a neoplastic phenotype; whereas, it induces apoptosis in non-neoplastic cells. [48] Persistent hCMV infection of tumor cells may lead to a selection of virus variants with changes in virus regulatory proteins that have lost their ability to induce cell cycle arrest. [63,64]

4. Escape of immune surveillance by cancer cells: Role of hCMV

Immunological tolerance is a process by which the immune system no longer recognizes an aberrant antigen as "foreign." [67] Through "natural" or "self-tolerance" the body does not mount an immune response to self-antigens. "Induced tolerance" to external antigens can be created by manipulating the immune system. Mechanisms of tolerance that exist to prevent autoimmune disease may also preclude the development of an adequate antitumor response. [65-67] This concept of "immune tolerance" may be particularly important in malignancies whose etiology is associated with inflammation. [68] Expression of hCMV proteins by infected tumor cells may induce 'immune tolerance' to tumor cells. Also, several tumor-derived factors contribute to the emergence of complex local and regional immunosuppressive networks, including VEGF, IL-10, TGF-β, and prostaglandin E-2 (PGE2). [66,69]

hCMV has evolved multiple strategies for immune evasion resulting in persistent viral infection in the host [70-74] Several hCMV proteins, including those expressed with IE genes, block the host cell MHC class I antigen expression, which is essential for activation of CD8+ T-lymphocyte anti-tumor cytotoxicity. hCMV UL83 protein (pp65) blocks antigen presentation of hCMV epitopes to CD8+ T-cells, and expression of hCMV UL18, a MHC class I homologue, disrupts "natural killer" (NK) cell recognition of hCMV-infected cells. [75] Disruption of hCMV antigen presentation by infected cells is mediated by hCMV protein US3, which sequesters MHC class I complexes in the endoplasmic reticulum, and hCMV protein US11 which causes dislocation of the MHC class I heavy chain from the cytoplasm. [76-78] hCMV-encoded IL-10 homologue impairs tumor antigen presentation by inhibiting maturation, normal differentiation and cytokine production of dendritic cells and macrophages.. [79-81] hCMV induces integrin $\alpha_v\beta_6$ expression in endothelial cells of blood vessels in different tissues, causing activation of TGF-β1, resulting in interference of host immune responses against tumor cells by blocking the activation of lymphocytes and monocyte derived phagocytes. [82] These direct immune-modulatory effects of hCMV on myeloid cells within the tumor microenvironment, along with expression of immunosuppressive cytokines provide a virtually impassable environment for the host anti-tumor immune system.

5. Influence of CMV on tumor microenvironment

Persistent hCMV infection of non-neoplastic cells in the tumor microenvironment leads to a paracrine secretion of inflammatory molecules that promote malignancy. [83] The secretome of hCMV-infected fibroblasts contains exceedingly high levels of growth factors, matrix remodeling proteins such as matrix metalloproteinases (MMPs), and angiogenic factors that signal through the TGF-β pathway. [47,84] These paracrine-secreted factors are also able to activate latent growth factors. PDGFs acts as strong mitogens and their overexpression is important in the pathogenesis of multiple malignancies. [85-87] In addition to growth factors, high levels of many ECM modifiers such as MMPs, tissue inhibitors of metalloproteinases (TIMPs) and urokinase receptor (uPAR) secreted by hCMV infected cells aiding, tumor invasion and metastasis. [84]

6. DNA mutations, impaired DNA repair mechanisms and epigenetic changes by hCMV that leads to genomic instability

hCMV infection can drive neoplastic transformation by causing chromosome damage and genetic instability in infected cells, particularly in vulnerable adult stem cells. [88-90] hCMV in combination with cytotoxic chemotherapy agents synergistically increases genotoxic effects. [91,92] The virus can induce specific chromosome 1 strand breaks at positions 1q42 and 1q21 in a replication-independent fashion, both of which are associated with DNA repair and replication genes. [89,93,94] hCMV IE1-72 and IE2-86 proteins when in conjunction with other viral oncogenic proteins (e.g., adenovirus E1A protein) that disrupt cell cycle can induce oncogenic transformation. [29]

hCMV can contribute to genomic instability through a variety of different pathways. In brief, the virus may induce chromosomal aberrations (e.g., production of micronuclei, misaligned chromosomes, chromosomal lagging and bridging) by hCMV UL76 protein. [95,96] The virus can also disrupt DNA repair pathways, including the activity of ATM and ATM-Rad3 (ATR). [97] More recently, hCMV has been shown to modulate oncogenesis through the telomerase pathway by activating human telomerase reverse transcriptase (hTERT) in fibroblasts and malignant cells. [98]

7. Conclusions

Significant advances have been made in understanding the roles of chronic inflammation, tumor microenvironment, cancer stem cells, tumor immunology, and infectious agents in the pathobiology of cancer. Several clinical and experimental findings suggest that hCMV may play a role in promoting certain cancers. In cells that are persistently infected with hCMV, the expression of viral proteins may prevent the immune system from identifying or removing these cells, thereby offsetting immune detection of transformed cells. The effects of hCMV in promoting tumor cell immune evasion may prove important in development of cancer immunotherapies, particularly if the hCMV-infected cells are resistant to the action of cytolytic peptides released by activated NK and cytotoxic T-cells. Also, if viral proteins that inhibit apoptosis are expressed by hCMV infected tumour cells, the cancer cells may be less susceptible conventional chemotherapeutic agents. Whether hCMV is ultimately established as an oncogenic virus will require additional research in the areas of virology, epidemiology and molecular oncology, and systematic refinement of the concept of "oncomodulation." Insights into the role of hCMV in oncogenesis may increase understanding of cancer biology and promote development of novel therapeutic strategies.

Author details

Prakash Vishnu[1] and David M. Aboulafia[1,2*]

*Address all correspondence to: david.aboulafia@vmmc.org

1 Floyd & Delores Jones Cancer Institute at Virginia Mason Medical Center, Seattle, WA, USA

2 Division of Hematology, University of Washington, Seattle, WA, USA

References

[1] Cinatl J, Scholz M, Kotchetkov R, Vogel JU, Doerr HW. Molecular mechanisms of the modulatory effects of HCMV infection in tumor cell biology. *Trends in molecular medicine.* Jan 2004;10(1):19-23.

[2] Harkins LE, Matlaf LA, Soroceanu L, et al. Detection of human cytomegalovirus in normal and neoplastic breast epithelium. *Herpesviridae.* 2010;1(1):8.

[3] Cobbs CS, Harkins L, Samanta M, et al. Human cytomegalovirus infection and expression in human malignant glioma. *Cancer research.* Jun 15 2002;62(12):3347-3350.

[4] Cobbs CS, Soroceanu L, Denham S, et al. Human cytomegalovirus induces cellular tyrosine kinase signaling and promotes glioma cell invasiveness. *Journal of neuro-oncology.* Dec 2007;85(3):271-280.

[5] Giuliani L, Jaxmar T, Casadio C, et al. Detection of oncogenic viruses SV40, BKV, JCV, HCMV, HPV and p53 codon 72 polymorphism in lung carcinoma. *Lung Cancer.* Sep 2007;57(3):273-281.

[6] Harkins L, Volk AL, Samanta M, et al. Specific localisation of human cytomegalovirus nucleic acids and proteins in human colorectal cancer. *Lancet.* Nov 16 2002;360(9345):1557-1563.

[7] Scheurer ME, Bondy ML, Aldape KD, Albrecht T, El-Zein R. Detection of human cytomegalovirus in different histological types of gliomas. *Acta neuropathologica.* Jul 2008;116(1):79-86.

[8] Castillo JP, Kowalik TF. HCMV infection: modulating the cell cycle and cell death. *International reviews of immunology.* Jan-Apr 2004;23(1-2):113-139.

[9] Hanahan D, Weinberg RA. Hallmarks of cancer: the next generation. *Cell.* Mar 4 2011;144(5):646-674.

[10] Colotta F, Allavena P, Sica A, Garlanda C, Mantovani A. Cancer-related inflammation, the seventh hallmark of cancer: links to genetic instability. *Carcinogenesis.* Jul 2009;30(7):1073-1081.

[11] Berasain C, Castillo J, Perugorria MJ, Latasa MU, Prieto J, Avila MA. Inflammation and liver cancer: new molecular links. *Annals of the New York Academy of Sciences.* Feb 2009;1155:206-221.

[12] Young LS, Rickinson AB. Epstein-Barr virus: 40 years on. *Nature reviews. Cancer.* Oct 2004;4(10):757-768.

[13] Schetter AJ, Heegaard NH, Harris CC. Inflammation and cancer: interweaving microRNA, free radical, cytokine and p53 pathways. *Carcinogenesis.* Jan 2010;31(1): 37-49.

[14] Hussain SP, Harris CC. Inflammation and cancer: an ancient link with novel potentials. *International journal of cancer. Journal international du cancer.* Dec 1 2007;121(11): 2373-2380.

[15] de Visser KE, Eichten A, Coussens LM. Paradoxical roles of the immune system during cancer development. *Nature reviews. Cancer.* Jan 2006;6(1):24-37.

[16] Grivennikov SI, Greten FR, Karin M. Immunity, inflammation, and cancer. *Cell.* Mar 19 2010;140(6):883-899.

[17] Balkwill F, Charles KA, Mantovani A. Smoldering and polarized inflammation in the initiation and promotion of malignant disease. *Cancer cell.* Mar 2005;7(3):211-217.

[18] Allavena P, Sica A, Garlanda C, Mantovani A. The Yin-Yang of tumor-associated macrophages in neoplastic progression and immune surveillance. *Immunological reviews.* Apr 2008;222:155-161.

[19] Zamarron BF, Chen W. Dual roles of immune cells and their factors in cancer development and progression. *International journal of biological sciences.* 2011;7(5):651-658.

[20] Gomez GG, Kruse CA. Mechanisms of malignant glioma immune resistance and sources of immunosuppression. *Gene therapy & molecular biology.* 2006;10(A):133-146.

[21] Wolf AM, Wolf D, Steurer M, Gastl G, Gunsilius E, Grubeck-Loebenstein B. Increase of regulatory T cells in the peripheral blood of cancer patients. *Clinical cancer research : an official journal of the American Association for Cancer Research.* Feb 2003;9(2): 606-612.

[22] Greten FR, Eckmann L, Greten TF, et al. IKKbeta links inflammation and tumorigenesis in a mouse model of colitis-associated cancer. *Cell.* Aug 6 2004;118(3):285-296.

[23] Cobbs CS, Brenman JE, Aldape KD, Bredt DS, Israel MA. Expression of nitric oxide synthase in human central nervous system tumors. *Cancer research.* Feb 15 1995;55(4): 727-730.

[24] Hara A, Okayasu I. Cyclooxygenase-2 and inducible nitric oxide synthase expression in human astrocytic gliomas: correlation with angiogenesis and prognostic significance. *Acta neuropathologica.* Jul 2004;108(1):43-48.

[25] Jia W, Jackson-Cook C, Graf MR. Tumor-infiltrating, myeloid-derived suppressor cells inhibit T cell activity by nitric oxide production in an intracranial rat glioma + vaccination model. *Journal of neuroimmunology.* Jun 2010;223(1-2):20-30.

[26] Cinatl J, Jr., Cinatl J, Vogel JU, Rabenau H, Kornhuber B, Doerr HW. Modulatory effects of human cytomegalovirus infection on malignant properties of cancer cells. *Intervirology.* 1996;39(4):259-269.

[27] Geder L, Sanford EJ, Rohner TJ, Rapp F. Cytomegalovirus and cancer of the prostate: in vitro transformation of human cells. *Cancer treatment reports.* Mar-Apr 1977;61(2): 139-146.

[28] Sanford EJ, Geder L, Laychock A, Rohner TJ, Jr., Rapp F. Evidence for the association of cytomegalovirus with carcinoma of the prostate. *The Journal of urology.* Nov 1977;118(5):789-792.

[29] Shen Y, Zhu H, Shenk T. Human cytomagalovirus IE1 and IE2 proteins are mutagenic and mediate "hit-and-run" oncogenic transformation in cooperation with the ade-

novirus E1A proteins. *Proceedings of the National Academy of Sciences of the United States of America.* Apr 1 1997;94(7):3341-3345.

[30] Plati J, Bucur O, Khosravi-Far R. Dysregulation of apoptotic signaling in cancer: molecular mechanisms and therapeutic opportunities. *Journal of cellular biochemistry.* Jul 1 2008;104(4):1124-1149.

[31] Pucci B, Kasten M, Giordano A. Cell cycle and apoptosis. *Neoplasia.* Jul-Aug 2000;2(4):291-299.

[32] Zhu H, Shen Y, Shenk T. Human cytomegalovirus IE1 and IE2 proteins block apoptosis. *Journal of virology.* Dec 1995;69(12):7960-7970.

[33] McCormick AL. Control of apoptosis by human cytomegalovirus. *Current topics in microbiology and immunology.* 2008;325:281-295.

[34] Michaelis M, Kotchetkov R, Vogel JU, Doerr HW, Cinatl J, Jr. Cytomegalovirus infection blocks apoptosis in cancer cells. *Cellular and molecular life sciences : CMLS.* Jun 2004;61(11):1307-1316.

[35] Skaletskaya A, Bartle LM, Chittenden T, McCormick AL, Mocarski ES, Goldmacher VS. A cytomegalovirus-encoded inhibitor of apoptosis that suppresses caspase-8 activation. *Proceedings of the National Academy of Sciences of the United States of America.* Jul 3 2001;98(14):7829-7834.

[36] Goldmacher VS, Bartle LM, Skaletskaya A, et al. A cytomegalovirus-encoded mitochondria-localized inhibitor of apoptosis structurally unrelated to Bcl-2. *Proceedings of the National Academy of Sciences of the United States of America.* Oct 26 1999;96(22): 12536-12541.

[37] Cinatl J, Jr., Cinatl J, Vogel JU, et al. Persistent human cytomegalovirus infection induces drug resistance and alteration of programmed cell death in human neuroblastoma cells. *Cancer research.* Jan 15 1998;58(2):367-372.

[38] Soroceanu L, Akhavan A, Cobbs CS. Platelet-derived growth factor-alpha receptor activation is required for human cytomegalovirus infection. *Nature.* Sep 18 2008;455(7211):391-395.

[39] Johnson RA, Wang X, Ma XL, Huong SM, Huang ES. Human cytomegalovirus upregulates the phosphatidylinositol 3-kinase (PI3-K) pathway: inhibition of PI3-K activity inhibits viral replication and virus-induced signaling. *Journal of virology.* Jul 2001;75(13):6022-6032.

[40] Johnson RA, Huong SM, Huang ES. Activation of the mitogen-activated protein kinase p38 by human cytomegalovirus infection through two distinct pathways: a novel mechanism for activation of p38. *Journal of virology.* Feb 2000;74(3):1158-1167.

[41] Kopfstein L, Christofori G. Metastasis: cell-autonomous mechanisms versus contributions by the tumor microenvironment. *Cellular and molecular life sciences : CMLS.* Feb 2006;63(4):449-468.

[42] Cruz-Monserrate Z, O'Connor KL. Integrin alpha 6 beta 4 promotes migration, invasion through Tiam1 upregulation, and subsequent Rac activation. *Neoplasia.* May 2008;10(5):408-417.

[43] Hall CL, Dubyk CW, Riesenberger TA, Shein D, Keller ET, van Golen KL. Type I collagen receptor (alpha2beta1) signaling promotes prostate cancer invasion through RhoC GTPase. *Neoplasia.* Aug 2008;10(8):797-803.

[44] Blaheta RA, Weich E, Marian D, et al. Human cytomegalovirus infection alters PC3 prostate carcinoma cell adhesion to endothelial cells and extracellular matrix. *Neoplasia.* Oct 2006;8(10):807-816.

[45] Blaheta RA, Beecken WD, Engl T, et al. Human cytomegalovirus infection of tumor cells downregulates NCAM (CD56): a novel mechanism for virus-induced tumor invasiveness. *Neoplasia.* Jul-Aug 2004;6(4):323-331.

[46] Goon PK, Lip GY, Boos CJ, Stonelake PS, Blann AD. Circulating endothelial cells, endothelial progenitor cells, and endothelial microparticles in cancer. *Neoplasia.* Feb 2006;8(2):79-88.

[47] Dumortier J, Streblow DN, Moses AV, et al. Human cytomegalovirus secretome contains factors that induce angiogenesis and wound healing. *Journal of virology.* Jul 2008;82(13):6524-6535.

[48] Maussang D, Verzijl D, van Walsum M, et al. Human cytomegalovirus-encoded chemokine receptor US28 promotes tumorigenesis. *Proceedings of the National Academy of Sciences of the United States of America.* Aug 29 2006;103(35):13068-13073.

[49] Reinhardt B, Mertens T, Mayr-Beyrle U, et al. HCMV infection of human vascular smooth muscle cells leads to enhanced expression of functionally intact PDGF beta-receptor. *Cardiovascular research.* Jul 1 2005;67(1):151-160.

[50] Kovacs A, Weber ML, Burns LJ, Jacob HS, Vercellotti GM. Cytoplasmic sequestration of p53 in cytomegalovirus-infected human endothelial cells. *The American journal of pathology.* Nov 1996;149(5):1531-1539.

[51] Murayama T, Mukaida N, Sadanari H, et al. The immediate early gene 1 product of human cytomegalovirus is sufficient for up-regulation of interleukin-8 gene expression. *Biochemical and biophysical research communications.* Dec 9 2000;279(1):298-304.

[52] Bentz GL, Yurochko AD. Human CMV infection of endothelial cells induces an angiogenic response through viral binding to EGF receptor and beta1 and beta3 integrins. *Proceedings of the National Academy of Sciences of the United States of America.* Apr 8 2008;105(14):5531-5536.

[53] Hsu SC, Volpert OV, Steck PA, et al. Inhibition of angiogenesis in human glioblastomas by chromosome 10 induction of thrombospondin-1. *Cancer research.* Dec 15 1996;56(24):5684-5691.

[54] Tenan M, Fulci G, Albertoni M, et al. Thrombospondin-1 is downregulated by anoxia and suppresses tumorigenicity of human glioblastoma cells. *The Journal of experimental medicine.* May 15 2000;191(10):1789-1798.

[55] Tsujii M, Kawano S, Tsuji S, Sawaoka H, Hori M, DuBois RN. Cyclooxygenase regulates angiogenesis induced by colon cancer cells. *Cell.* May 29 1998;93(5):705-716.

[56] Sanchez V, Spector DH. Subversion of cell cycle regulatory pathways. *Current topics in microbiology and immunology.* 2008;325:243-262.

[57] Jault FM, Jault JM, Ruchti F, et al. Cytomegalovirus infection induces high levels of cyclins, phosphorylated Rb, and p53, leading to cell cycle arrest. *Journal of virology.* Nov 1995;69(11):6697-6704.

[58] Salvant BS, Fortunato EA, Spector DH. Cell cycle dysregulation by human cytomegalovirus: influence of the cell cycle phase at the time of infection and effects on cyclin transcription. *Journal of virology.* May 1998;72(5):3729-3741.

[59] Song YJ, Stinski MF. Inhibition of cell division by the human cytomegalovirus IE86 protein: role of the p53 pathway or cyclin-dependent kinase 1/cyclin B1. *Journal of virology.* Feb 2005;79(4):2597-2603.

[60] Hume AJ, Finkel JS, Kamil JP, Coen DM, Culbertson MR, Kalejta RF. Phosphorylation of retinoblastoma protein by viral protein with cyclin-dependent kinase function. *Science.* May 9 2008;320(5877):797-799.

[61] Hwang ES, Zhang Z, Cai H, et al. Human cytomegalovirus IE1-72 protein interacts with p53 and inhibits p53-dependent transactivation by a mechanism different from that of IE2-86 protein. *Journal of virology.* Dec 2009;83(23):12388-12398.

[62] Luo MH, Fortunato EA. Long-term infection and shedding of human cytomegalovirus in T98G glioblastoma cells. *Journal of virology.* Oct 2007;81(19):10424-10436.

[63] Furukawa T. A variant of human cytomegalovirus derived from a persistently infected culture. *Virology.* Aug 1984;137(1):191-194.

[64] Ogura T, Tanaka J, Kamiya S, Sato H, Ogura H, Hatano M. Human cytomegalovirus persistent infection in a human central nervous system cell line: production of a variant virus with different growth characteristics. *The Journal of general virology.* Dec 1986;67 (Pt 12):2605-2616.

[65] Dunn GP, Bruce AT, Ikeda H, Old LJ, Schreiber RD. Cancer immunoediting: from immunosurveillance to tumor escape. *Nature immunology.* Nov 2002;3(11):991-998.

[66] Kim R, Emi M, Tanabe K. Cancer immunosuppression and autoimmune disease: beyond immunosuppressive networks for tumour immunity. *Immunology.* Oct 2006;119(2):254-264.

[67] Drake CG, Jaffee E, Pardoll DM. Mechanisms of immune evasion by tumors. *Advances in immunology.* 2006;90:51-81.

[68] Kamp DW, Shacter E, Weitzman SA. Chronic inflammation and cancer: the role of the mitochondria. *Oncology (Williston Park).* Apr 30 2011;25(5):400-410, 413.

[69] Kim R, Emi M, Tanabe K, Arihiro K. Tumor-driven evolution of immunosuppressive networks during malignant progression. *Cancer research.* Jun 1 2006;66(11):5527-5536.

[70] Hengel H, Brune W, Koszinowski UH. Immune evasion by cytomegalovirus--survival strategies of a highly adapted opportunist. *Trends in microbiology.* May 1998;6(5): 190-197.

[71] Loenen WA, Bruggeman CA, Wiertz EJ. Immune evasion by human cytomegalovirus: lessons in immunology and cell biology. *Seminars in immunology.* Feb 2001;13(1): 41-49.

[72] Michelson S. Human cytomegalovirus escape from immune detection. *Intervirology.* 1999;42(5-6):301-307.

[73] Scholz M, Doerr HW, Cinatl J. Human cytomegalovirus retinitis: pathogenicity, immune evasion and persistence. *Trends in microbiology.* Apr 2003;11(4):171-178.

[74] Wiertz E, Hill A, Tortorella D, Ploegh H. Cytomegaloviruses use multiple mechanisms to elude the host immune response. *Immunology letters.* Jun 1 1997;57(1-3): 213-216.

[75] Farrell HE, Vally H, Lynch DM, et al. Inhibition of natural killer cells by a cytomegalovirus MHC class I homologue in vivo. *Nature.* Apr 3 1997;386(6624):510-514.

[76] Greijer AE, Verschuuren EA, Dekkers CA, et al. Expression dynamics of human cytomegalovirus immune evasion genes US3, US6, and US11 in the blood of lung transplant recipients. *The Journal of infectious diseases.* Aug 1 2001;184(3):247-255.

[77] Benz C, Hengel H. MHC class I-subversive gene functions of cytomegalovirus and their regulation by interferons-an intricate balance. *Virus genes.* 2000;21(1-2):39-47.

[78] Besold K, Wills M, Plachter B. Immune evasion proteins gpUS2 and gpUS11 of human cytomegalovirus incompletely protect infected cells from CD8 T cell recognition. *Virology.* Aug 15 2009;391(1):5-19.

[79] Chang WL, Baumgarth N, Yu D, Barry PA. Human cytomegalovirus-encoded interleukin-10 homolog inhibits maturation of dendritic cells and alters their functionality. *Journal of virology.* Aug 2004;78(16):8720-8731.

[80] Cheeran MC, Hu S, Sheng WS, Peterson PK, Lokensgard JR. CXCL10 production from cytomegalovirus-stimulated microglia is regulated by both human and viral interleukin-10. *Journal of virology.* Apr 2003;77(8):4502-4515.

[81] Nachtwey J, Spencer JV. HCMV IL-10 suppresses cytokine expression in monocytes through inhibition of nuclear factor-kappaB. *Viral immunology.* Dec 2008;21(4): 477-482.

[82] Tabata T, Kawakatsu H, Maidji E, et al. Induction of an epithelial integrin alphavbeta6 in human cytomegalovirus-infected endothelial cells leads to activation of transforming growth factor-beta1 and increased collagen production. *The American journal of pathology.* Apr 2008;172(4):1127-1140.

[83] Chan G, Bivins-Smith ER, Smith MS, Smith PM, Yurochko AD. Transcriptome analysis reveals human cytomegalovirus reprograms monocyte differentiation toward an M1 macrophage. *J Immunol.* Jul 1 2008;181(1):698-711.

[84] Streblow DN, Dumortier J, Moses AV, Orloff SL, Nelson JA. Mechanisms of cytomegalovirus-accelerated vascular disease: induction of paracrine factors that promote angiogenesis and wound healing. *Current topics in microbiology and immunology.* 2008;325:397-415.

[85] Ahmad A, Wang Z, Kong D, et al. Platelet-derived growth factor-D contributes to aggressiveness of breast cancer cells by up-regulating Notch and NF-kappaB signaling pathways. *Breast cancer research and treatment.* Feb 2011;126(1):15-25.

[86] Campbell JS, Hughes SD, Gilbertson DG, et al. Platelet-derived growth factor C induces liver fibrosis, steatosis, and hepatocellular carcinoma. *Proceedings of the National Academy of Sciences of the United States of America.* Mar 1 2005;102(9):3389-3394.

[87] Shih AH, Holland EC. Platelet-derived growth factor (PDGF) and glial tumorigenesis. *Cancer letters.* Feb 8 2006;232(2):139-147.

[88] Hartmann M, Brunnemann H. Chromosome aberrations in cytomegalovirus-infected human diploid cell culture. *Acta virologica.* Mar 1972;16(2):176.

[89] Fortunato EA, Spector DH. Viral induction of site-specific chromosome damage. *Reviews in medical virology.* Jan-Feb 2003;13(1):21-37.

[90] Jefford CE, Irminger-Finger I. Mechanisms of chromosome instability in cancers. *Critical reviews in oncology/hematology.* Jul 2006;59(1):1-14.

[91] Deng CZ, AbuBakar S, Fons MP, Boldogh I, Albrecht T. Modulation of the frequency of human cytomegalovirus-induced chromosome aberrations by camptothecin. *Virology.* Jul 1992;189(1):397-401.

[92] Deng CZ, AbuBakar S, Fons MP, et al. Cytomegalovirus-enhanced induction of chromosome aberrations in human peripheral blood lymphocytes treated with potent genotoxic agents. *Environmental and molecular mutagenesis.* 1992;19(4):304-310.

[93] Fortunato EA, Dell'Aquila ML, Spector DH. Specific chromosome 1 breaks induced by human cytomegalovirus. *Proceedings of the National Academy of Sciences of the United States of America.* Jan 18 2000;97(2):853-858.

[94] Baumgartner M, Schneider R, Auer B, Herzog H, Schweiger M, Hirsch-Kauffmann M. Fluorescence in situ mapping of the human nuclear NAD+ ADP-ribosyltransferase gene (ADPRT) and two secondary sites to human chromosomal bands 1q42, 13q34, and 14q24. *Cytogenetics and cell genetics.* 1992;61(3):172-174.

[95] Albrecht T, Deng CZ, Abdel-Rahman SZ, Fons M, Cinciripini P, El-Zein RA. Differential mutagen sensitivity of peripheral blood lymphocytes from smokers and non-smokers: effect of human cytomegalovirus infection. *Environmental and molecular mutagenesis.* 2004;43(3):169-178.

[96] Siew VK, Duh CY, Wang SK. Human cytomegalovirus UL76 induces chromosome aberrations. *Journal of biomedical science.* 2009;16:107.

[97] Luo MH, Rosenke K, Czornak K, Fortunato EA. Human cytomegalovirus disrupts both ataxia telangiectasia mutated protein (ATM)- and ATM-Rad3-related kinase-mediated DNA damage responses during lytic infection. *Journal of virology.* Feb 2007;81(4):1934-1950.

[98] Straat K, Liu C, Rahbar A, et al. Activation of telomerase by human cytomegalovirus. *Journal of the National Cancer Institute.* Apr 1 2009;101(7):488-497.

[99] Michaelis M, Baumgarten P, Mittelbronn M, Driever PH, Doerr HW, Cinatl J, Jr. Oncomodulation by human cytomegalovirus: novel clinical findings open new roads. *Medical microbiology and immunology.* Feb 2011;200(1):1-5.

[100] Michaelis M, Doerr HW, Cinatl J. The story of human cytomegalovirus and cancer: increasing evidence and open questions. *Neoplasia.* Jan 2009;11(1):1-9.

Chapter 7

Cytomegalovirus Tegument Proteins and the Development of Novel Antiviral Therapeutics

John Paul III Tomtishen

Additional information is available at the end of the chapter

http://dx.doi.org/10.5772/55156

1. Introduction

Cytomegalovirus (CMV) is a widespread pathogen that infects a majority of the world's population by early adulthood with approximately 50-85% of individuals over 40 being seropositive [1,2]. CMV can establish a life-long infection with its host by becoming latent during the lysogenic stage of the viral life cycle in which the virus becomes dormant and the shedding and production of infectious virions ceases [3]. However, the virus can later re-enter the lytic stage of the viral life cycle when presented with certain environmental cues, such as stress, thereby triggering the production of viral progeny and resulting in an acute infection of the host. Immunocompetent individuals generally display no symptoms of acute CMV infection, but CMV can cause morbidity and mortality in those with weakened or not fully developed immune systems [4]. The clinical manifestations of CMV infections in those with weakened immune systems, include spiking fever, malaise, leucopenia, encephalitis, pneumonitis, hepatitis, uveitis, retinitis, gastrointestinal disease and graft rejection [5,6]. If primary infection or reactivation of CMV occurs during pregnancy in women, serious complications will arise for the fetus or developing embryo. CMV is the leading cause of viral birth defects, including microcephaly, mental retardation, spastic paralysis, hepatosplenomegaly, anemia, thrombocytopenia, deafness, and optic nerve atrophy that subsequently leads to blindness [5, 7]. CMV is also responsible for 8% of infectious mononucleosis cases [8].

Although immunocompetent individuals generally display no symptoms of CMV infection, CMV has been implicated in playing a role in several proliferative and inflammatory diseases [9]. CMV has been linked with several forms of cancer, such as colon, breast, and prostate. Previously, CMV was regarded as having an oncomodulatory role in cancers by infecting tumor cells and modulating their malignant properties. It was hypothesized that tumor cells provided a genetic environment that allowed CMV to exert its oncomodulatory effects. CMV was then identified as a potential therapeutic target in those tumors infected with CMV [10-12]. However, recent evidence supports oncogenic properties of CMV in certain cancers, such those as in salivary gland [13]. Furthermore, epidemiological and pathological studies suggest a strong link between CMV and atherosclerosis [9]. A potential mechanism for CMV in the pathogenesis of atherosclerosis involves the reactivation of virus followed by virus-induced enhancement of vascular inflammation and damage through smooth cell proliferation, uptake of low-density lipoproteins, and narrowing of the vessel lumen [1].

Antiviral agents that inhibit CMV viral replication exist, including ganciclovir, valganciclovir (the prodrug of ganciclovir), foscarnet, and cidofovir [1]. The primary mechanism of action of ganciclovir/valganciclovir against CMV is through the inhibition of the replication of viral DNA by ganciclovir-5′-triphosphate, which includes a selective and potent inhibition of the viral DNA polymerase [14]. Foscarnet, by comparison, interferes with the exchange of pyrophosphate from deoxynucleoside triphosphate during viral replication by binding to a site on the CMV DNA polymerase [15]. Similarly, cidofovir inhibits CMV DNA synthesis by DNA chain termination following incorporation of two consecutive cidofovir molecules at the 3'-end of the DNA chain [16]. Nonetheless, the antiviral agents commonly used to treat CMV infections suffer from high hematologic, renal, and neutropenia toxicity, low bioavailability and the development of drug-resistant virus strains [9,17]. Furthermore, there is no effective vaccine available.

The lack of an effective treatment for CMV infections has increased interest in the identification of targets for the development of novel CMV antiviral treatments. These include proteins found within the tegument of CMV virions. These proteins are abundant and play pivotal roles in the viral life cycle, including immune evasion, viral entry, gene expression, assembly of new virus particles and egress through an envelopment-deenvelopment-reenvelopment process [18]. The structure of the CMV tegument, the roles of some major tegument proteins in the CMV life cycle, and the therapeutic potential of CMV tegument proteins will be reviewed.

2. Cytomegalovirus structure and function of the tegument

CMV is a member of the *Betaherpesvirinae* sub-family of the *Herpesviridae* family, (Figure 1). The virion has an icosahedral protein nucleocapsid that contains the 235-kb double-stranded DNA. The capsid is surrounded by a proteinaceous tegument and an outer lipid envelope [1]. CMV virions gain entry into a host cell via a membrane fusion event involving the outer membrane of the cell and the glycoproteins located on the lipid envelope of the virion. When the cell membrane and lipid envelope fuse, the DNA-containing protein nucleocapsid and tegument proteins are released into the host cell. This initiates the lytic stage of the viral life cycle [19].

The proteins in the tegument are excellent candidates for novel CMV antiviral treatments due to their abundance and significant roles in all stages of the viral life cycle. The tegument, located between the outer lipid membrane and the icosahedral protein nucleocapsid is largely unstructured and amorphous although some structuring is seen with the binding of tegument

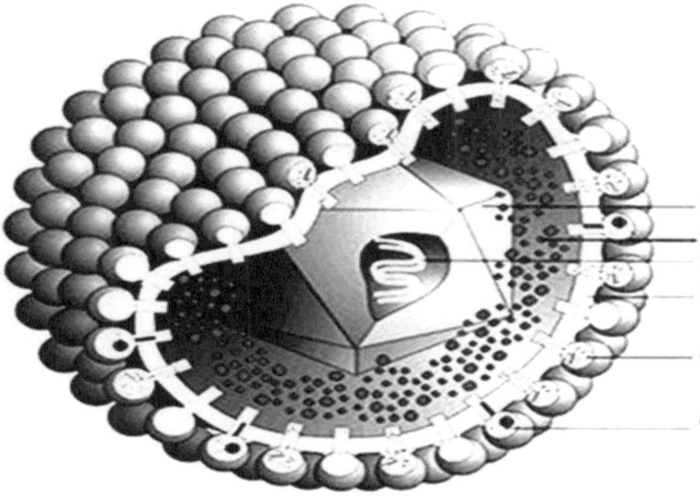

Figure 1. A cartoon depicting the structure of the HCMV virion. (Image obtained from (http://www.virology.net/big_virology/bvdnaherpes.html website) courtesy of Dr. Marko Reschke in Marburg, Germany).

proteins to the protein capsid [20]. The tegument proteins comprise more than half of the total proteins found within infectious CMV virions [21]. Tegument proteins are phosphorylated and undergo other posttranslational modifications, but the significance of these modifications is unknown [19]. A common biochemical sequence to direct proteins into the tegument has not been identified, and the process of assembling the viral tegument upon viral egress and disassembly upon viral entry into cells is unclear [22]. Incorporation of proteins in the tegument is likely facilitated by the phosphorylation of the tegument proteins, their subcellular localization to the assembly site and their interaction with capsids or the cytoplasmic tails of envelope proteins [18].

As mentioned, the tegument proteins gain entry into the host cell along with the DNA-containing protein nucleocapsid upon fusion of the outer membrane of the host cell and the outer glycoprotein riddled lipid membrane of the CMV virion [19]. Once the tegument proteins are released into the cytoplasm, they become functionally active and participate in all stages of the viral life cycle [1].

3. Cytomegalovirus tegument proteins

The CMV tegument proteins play pivotal roles illustrated in Figure 2. The known or inferred functions of tegument proteins are presented in Table 1, compiled using a functional profiling of the CMV genome from a global mutational analysis [18,62,63]. Gene expression classifications are based on when expression occurs during the viral life cycle (Immediate-Early, Early, Early-Late, and Late). Finally, the tegument proteins are categorized based on their role in lytic replication. Some proteins are essential for replication, while others are required for efficient replication (augmentative), or dispensable for lytic replication. The roles of major tegument proteins are presented in sections 3.1-3.4 in the context of the various stages of the CMV life cycle, which includes viral entry, viral replication and gene expression, immune evasion of the host, and assembly and egress of new infectious virions.

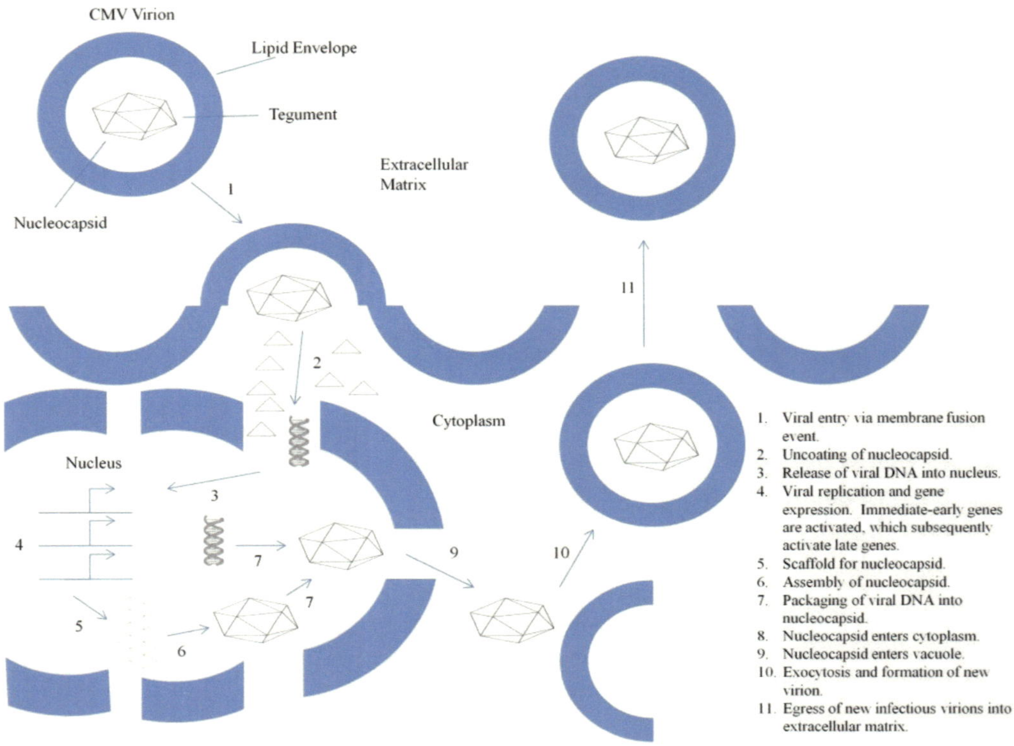

Figure 2. Illustration of the CMV life cycle from viral entry to egress of new infectious virions.

3.1. Viral entry

Mechanistically, the CMV virions enter host cells through a membrane fusion event involving the host cell's outer membrane and the glycoproteins located on the lipid envelope of the CMV virions [19]. The receptors on the viral envelope connect to complementary receptors on the cell membrane of the host cell. This initial interaction makes the cell susceptible to further interactions that allow the membranes to fuse, and the subsequent disassembly and release of the viral genomic DNA and tegument into the host cell. It is believed that several tegument proteins mediate delivery of the DNA-containing nucleocapsid to the nuclear pore complex and the release of the viral DNA into the nucleus [18]. Comparisons with other herpesviruses suggest that the UL47 and UL48 CMV tegument proteins, along with microtubule motor proteins, facilitate the delivery of the CMV nucleocapsids to the nuclear pore complex and the release of the CMV genome into the nucleus [18,64]. Pp150 may also play a role in viral entry due to its tight association with the CMV capsids [65].

3.2. Viral replication and gene expression

Once the viral genome enters the nucleus of the host cell, the viral immediate-early genes are expressed through their activation by the pp71 tegument protein, which initiates the lytic stage of the viral life cycle and the subsequent replication of the 235-kb double-stranded CMV DNA genome [46]. It is important to note though that the expression of the immediate-early genes can be repressed resulting in a latent infection that is characterized by the minimization of viral gene expression and the inhibition of the assembly and egress of new viral progeny [1,66]. Although pp71 is known to play a pivotal role in the expression of the immediate-early genes during the lytic stage of the CMV life cycle, the gene products of UL35 and UL69 have been implicated in gene expression [18]. However, more research is necessary to identify the other tegument proteins involved in viral gene expression.

3.3. Immune evasion

CMV evades the host cell immune system through the targeting of intrinsic, innate, and adaptive immune responses by several different tegument proteins, including pp65, pp71, and IRS1/TRS1. pp65 the major tegument protein involved in immune evasion of the host as well as IRS1/TRS1 modulate the innate and adaptive immune responses. pp71 modulates the intrinsic immune defense through its neutralization of the Daxx-mediated repression of immediate-early gene expression. Without immune evasion, the lytic stage of the viral life cycle is inhibited. The roles of pp65 and pp71 in modulating the host cell immune response is further discussed below in sections 4.1 and 4.3 respectively [18].

3.4. Assembly and egress

After viral DNA replication, the immediate-early gene products, which include several tegument proteins as seen in Table 1, turn on the expression of viral late genes [1]. The viral late proteins are mainly structural components that assist in the assembly and egress of newly formed infectious CMV virions [1]. The primary tegument proteins involved in assembly and egress are pp150, pp28, and UL97. pp150 directs the movement of the cytoplasmic capsids to the site for particle formation, while pp28 directs the enclosure of the tegument proteins and DNA-containing nucleocapsids within an enveloped particle [18,26,52]. UL97 phosphorylates the tegument proteins through its kinase activity, which may facilitate the incorporation of the tegument proteins into new infectious virions [18,30]. Once the virions are packaged, they are shed from the host cell through an exocytosis mechanism which uses the host cell's transport system to enclose vacuoles containing the newly synthesized infectious virions for release into the extracellular space.

Gene (Protein)	Expression	Essential for Lytic Replication	Known or Inferred Function	Reference
UL23	Early-Late	Dispensable	Involved in events immediately after virus penetration	[23]
UL24	Early-Late	Dispensable	Involved in events immediately after virus penetration	[23]
UL25	Late	Dispensable	Structural protein	[25]
UL26	Early-Late	Augmentative	Transcriptional activation	[24]
UL32 (pp150)	Late	Essential	Virion egress (directs capsid to the site of final envelopment)	[26]
UL35	Late	Augmentative	Viral replication and particle formation	[27]
UL36	Immediate-Early	Dispensable	Control of a caspase-independent cell death pathway	[28]
UL38	Immediate-Early	Augmentative	Control of apoptosis	[29]
UL43	Late	Dispensable	Involved in events immediately after virus penetration	[23]
UL44	Early	Essential	CMV DNA polymerase processivity/transcription factor	[31]
UL45	Late	Augmentative	Influences virus growth at low multiplicities of infection	[32]
UL47	Late	Augmentative	Release of viral DNA from nucleocapsid Disassembling of virus particles	[33]
UL48	Late	Essential	Deubiquitinating protease Release of viral DNA from capsid	[34]
UL50	Early	Essential	Egress of nucleocapsids	[35]
UL53	Late	Essential	Egress of nucleocapsids	[36]
UL54	Early	Essential	CMV DNA polymerase	[37]
UL56	Early-Late	Dispensable	DNA packaging	[38]
UL57	Early	Essential	Single-stranded DNA-binding protein	[39]
UL69	Early-Late	Augmentative	Nuclear export of unspliced mRNAs Arrests cell cycle in G1 phase	[40]
UL71	Early-Late	Augmentative/ Essential	Late envelopment	[41]
UL72	Late	Dispensable	Inactive	[42]
UL76	Early	Augmentative/ Essential	Modulation of gene expression	[43]

http://dx.doi.org/10.5772/55156

Gene (Protein)	Expression	Essential for Lytic Replication	Known or Inferred Function	Reference
UL77	Early	Essential	DNA packaging/cleavage	[44]
UL79	Early-Late	Essential	Promotes the accumulation of late viral transcripts	[45]
UL82 (pp71)	Immediate-Early	Augmentative	Degrades Daxx; facilitates Immediate-Early gene expression	[46]
UL83 (pp65)	Early-Late	Dispensable	Endogenous kinase activity Associated kinase activity Evasion of adaptive immunity Evasion of innate immunity	[47,58,59]
UL84	Early	Essential	CMV DNA replication	[48]
UL88	Late	Dispensable	Unknown	N/A
UL93	Late	Essential	Virion packaging	[49]
UL94	Late	Augmentative/ Essential	Putative DNA-binding protein	[50]
UL96	Early	Augmentative/ Essential	Preserves the integrity of the nucleocapsid during translocation from the nucleus to the cytoplasm	[51]
UL97	Early-Late	Augmentative	Kinase that phosphorylates UL44 Stimulates DNA replication, assembly, and egress Cyclin-dependent kinase-like functions	[30,60,61]
UL99 (pp28)	Late	Essential	Directs the enclosure of enveloped virus particles	[52]
UL103	Late	Augmentative	Regulates virus particle and dense body egress	[53]
UL112	Early	Augmentative	CMV DNA replication	[54]
IRS1/TRS1	Early-Late	Augmentative/ Essential	Inhibits PKR antiviral response Virion assembly	[55]
US22	Early	Dispensable	Involved in events immediately after virus penetration	[23]
US23	Early	Augmentative	Colocalization with pp65	[57]
US24	Early	Augmentative	Activation of viral gene expression	[56]

Table 1. CMV tegument proteins and their known or inferred function.

4. Cytomegalovirus tegument proteins as potential antiviral targets

Since the CMV tegument proteins play pivotal roles in all stages of the lytic stage of the viral life cycle, they are candidates for novel antiviral treatments. An antiviral agent able to bind to a major tegument protein and inhibit its function would prevent CMV from replicating its viral DNA genome and producing new infectious virions. This would have great therapeutic value. Examples of how tegument proteins could be targeted therapeutically are presented below (See Figure 3).

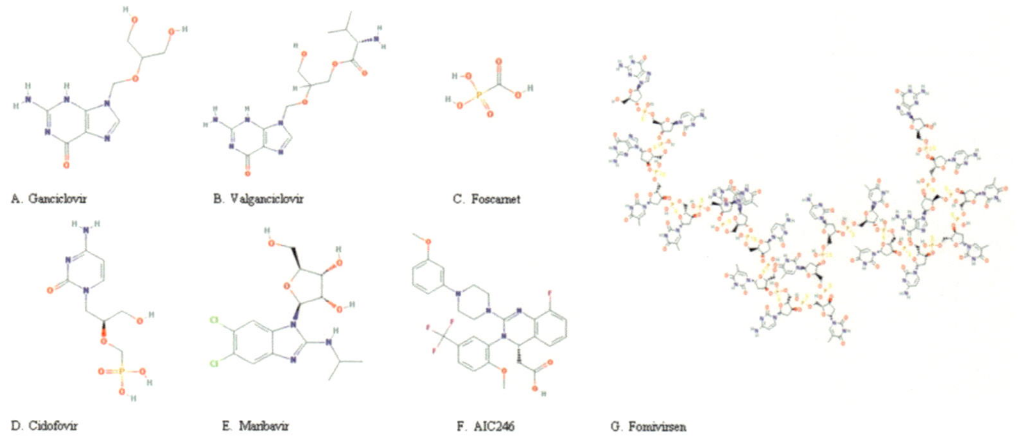

Figure 3. Current and developmental antiviral agents that target acute CMV infection.

4.1. pp65

A good tegument protein to target would be pp65, since it is the most abundant tegument protein [67]. pp65 is implicated in counteracting both innate and adaptive immune responses during CMV infections. It invokes humoral and cellular immunity and is the dominant target antigen of cytotoxic T lymphocytes [67]. In addition to pp65 being antigenic, it can also be considered a good antiviral target due to its immunomodulatory role. pp65 prevents immediate-early proteins from being recognized by components of the immune system in addition to inhibiting the synthesis of the various components involved in the host cell's immune response through its associated enzymatic kinase activity [58,59]. Thus, if you can inhibit the function of pp65, the host cell immune response would be able to inhibit the CMV viral life cycle.

Recent evidence in support of pp65 as a target for a novel antiviral treatment strategy concerns its subcellular localization during the lytic stage of the viral life cycle. pp65 migrates to the nucleoli at the early stages of infection, which suggests a functional relationship between its localization and the lytic stage of the viral life cycle [68]. However, pp65 begins to migrate to the cytoplasm 48 hours into the lytic cycle through cyclin-dependent kinase activity and a Crm 1 exporter mediated migration [69,70]. It is likely that pp65 does not migrate independently to the nucleoli as it remains in the cytoplasm in the absence of other components of CMV [71, 72]. This is significant as the localization patterns of the tegument proteins are correlated with their function [73]. Furthermore, pp65 has a bipartite nuclear localization signal, which implies that the nuclear localization signal is in a region that is initially inaccessible to importin proteins

[74]. Another tegument protein may bind to pp65,, inducing a conformational change that allows the inaccessible nuclear localization signal to be recognized by nuclear transport molecules, triggering the characteristic nuclear localization of pp65 and the initiation of the lytic cycle [71,72]. Importantly pp65 co-localizes with the tegument protein associated with the CMV US23 gene product [57]. Thus, the US23 gene product could be the other tegument protein necessary for pp65 to enter the nucleoli (also see section 4.2 UL97). Thus, two monoclonal antibodies could be developed to target antigens present on the surfaces of pp65 and the US23 gene product, which would prevent them from interacting and inhibit the development of the lytic stage of the CMV life cycle.

Additionally, pp65 can also be used to develop a vaccine to prevent or inhibit CMV infection. An excellent example of pp65 being utilized to develop a novel vaccine to prevent CMV infection concerns the two plasmid DNA vaccine, ASP0113. Currently, ASP0113 is in Phase I/II clinical trials to prevent CMV infection in solid organ transplant recipients at high risk for CMV infection. The vaccine is comprised of the highly immunogenic pp65 tegument protein and the gB CMV surface protein, which utilizes the ability of pp65 to induce cell-mediated response and gB to induce humoral immune system responses in those infected with CMV. Results show a reduction in the number of CMV episodes and the time to initial viremia [75].

4.2. UL97

The UL97 gene product is also a tegument protein that could be targeted for the development of a novel antiviral therapeutic. UL97 stimulates DNA replication, assembly, and egress in addition to being a known kinase homologue [30,76]. UL97's kinase activity makes CMV susceptible to the current CMV antiviral ganciclovir, a synthetic 2'-deoxy-guanosine analogue. UL97 phosphorylates this synthetic analog to a deoxyguanosine triphosphate analogue, which competitively inhibits the incorporation of it by viral DNA polymerase. This competitive inhibition results in the termination of CMV DNA elongation [77].

Currently, a specific inhibitor of UL97 protein kinase activity, maribavir, inhibits viral replication and is in clinical trials [78]. Maribavir is a benzimidazole riboside and inhibits CMV DNA assembly as well as the egress of CMV nucleocapsids from infected host cells [78]. Maribavir was given fast track status by the Food and Drug Administration and is being investigated in Phase 2 clinical trials using a high dose treatment option for clinically significant CMV viremia.

The UL97 gene product also shows due to its association with pp65. UL97 and pp65 act directly to form a complex during viral replication. When UL97 is genetically ablated or pharmacologically inhibited, pp65 localizes in unusual refractile bodies, which suggests that UL97 is essential for the successful localization of pp65 to the nucleus of the host cell at the beginning of the lytic stage of the viral life cycle [79]. Similarly to US23, UL97 may direct pp65 into the nucleus to initiate the lytic stage of CMV replication [71,72]. Furthermore, a pp65 deletion mutant exhibits modest resistance to maribavir [80]. pp65 may negatively regulate UL97 by sequestering kinase that would be available to promote viral replication [81]. The interaction between pp65 and UL97 could influence pp65-mediated immune evasion, because the presentation of viral immediate-early proteins to T cells is blocked when the proteins are phosphorylated by UL97 kinase [81,82].

4.3. pp71

pp71 is also a major target for CMV antiviral research as it influences the activation of immediate-early gene expression at the start of the lytic cycle [83]. Mechanistically, pp71 activates viral gene expression through the neutralization of the effects of the cellular Daxx protein, which is recruited to promoters by DNA-binding transcription factors, resulting in the repression of viral transcription [84]. pp71 binds to two inherent domains on Daxx and induces its proteasomal degradation [85]. pp71 is slows the intracellular transport of MHC class I molecules, which limits the display of CMV antigens on the surface of infected cells to cytotoxic T lymphocytes [86].

A UL82 gene deletion mutant may serve as a potential novel CMV vaccine candidate as it can enter cells efficiently and activate the innate immune response through interactions with cell surface receptors. However viral gene expression is disrupted during infection when cells are infected at a low multiplicity of the UL82 gene deletion mutant. The expression of the immediate-early genes that are involved in the host anti-viral response is blocked. One of the genes whose expression would be blocked is the immediate-early 2 (IE2) gene that can antagonize the host innate immune response by attenuating the interferon β response and blocking chemokine expression. If the expression of IE2 is blocked, the number of cytotoxic T lymphocytes and natural killer cells recruited to the infected cell would increase. Furthermore, viral replication is limited with low multiplicity of infection with the UL82 gene mutant as this would promote a robust anti-viral immune response. Thus, a novel antiviral treatment could target pp71 and its ability to control the activation of immediate-early gene expression [87].

4.4. Tegument structural proteins

The structural proteins of CMV with therapeutic potential include pp150, pp65 (above), pp28, pp38, and the gene products of UL55 and UL75, as they play pivotal roles in the CMV life cycle and are immunogenic. pp150, the second most abundant tegument protein behind pp65, plays a role in the assembly and egress of new infectious virus particles. It is necessary to incorporate nucleocapsids into these new infectious virus particles [21]. It is essential for maintaining the stability of the cytoplasmic capsids and directing their movement [1,88]. It also plays a role in the reorganization of the cytoplasmic assembly compartment during virion assembly [88]. pp28 is largely responsible for the cytoplasmic envelopment of tegument proteins and capsids during assembly and egress [89].

pp38 is a mitogen-activated protein kinase and has a critical function in CMV viral DNA replication. pp38 kinase activity is significantly increased after CMV infection, and inhibition of this kinase activity inhibits CMV-induced hyperphosphorylation of pRb and the phosphorylation of heat shock protein 27. This suggests that pp38 activation is involved in virus-mediated changes in host cell metabolism throughout the CMV infection [90].

http://dx.doi.org/10.5772/55156

The gene products of UL55 and UL75 by comparison have been shown to be involved Sp1 and NF-kappaB activation during the earliest stages of CMV infection via a cellular receptor-viral ligand interaction. This is based on the observation that the cellular transcription factors Sp1 and NF-kappaB are upregulated shortly after the binding of purified live or UV-inactivated CMV to the cell surface, which has also been seen in other systems where cellular factors are induced following a receptor-ligand interaction [91].

All tegument proteins elicit a strong humoral immune response [92]. This is significant, since the host immunological functions are clearly limit CMV-associated disease [93]. Novel therapeutics could take advantage of the highly immunogenic nature of the CMV structural proteins. Potentially, an antibody could be designed that recognizes the CMV antigens expressed on these proteins and could be exploited to deliver an active drug compound that can inhibit the lytic replication of the virus. This strategy is used to target certain cancers. Additionally, a monoclonal antibody could simply be used to help the immune system locate the CMV immunogenic structural proteins and end the CMV infection.

Additionally, structural phosphoproteins, such as pp65 and pp150, are good candidates for subunit vaccine development, since they elicit cytotoxic T lymphocyte responses. A CMV subunit vaccine would contain viral antigens without the CMV DNA genome. It would be less likely to cause adverse reactions and would be clinically valuable in view of the high hematologic and renal toxicity and low bioavailability of current antiviral treatments targeting acute CMV infection [94].

4.5. UL94

Although it is not critical for viral replication unlike the majority of potential CMV targets, UL94 could also be targeted by a novel antiviral agent. Studies of UL94 stop mutants show that UL94 plays a role in the secondary envelopment of viral particles. When the UL94 gene is absent or not functioning, the UL99 (pp28) tegument protein responsible for the cytoplasmic envelopment of tegument proteins during assembly and egress exhibits aberrant localization and there is a complete block of secondary envelopment of virions. Thus, UL94 functions late in the CMV lytic life cycle to direct pp28 to the assembly complex, facilitating the secondary envelopment of CMV virions [95].

If a molecule is able to target UL94 and inhibit its function, the assembly and egress of virion progeny will be blocked, since the secondary envelopment of CMV virions will not occur. A therapeutic targeting UL94 could utilize the interaction between UL94 and the pp28 structural protein. For example, a new antiviral could focus on the ability of pp28 to elicit a strong humoral immune response through the release of antibodies targeting the CMV specific immunoglobulin as mentioned above. Two monoclonal antibodies could also be developed to target pp28 and UL94 that could inhibit UL94 from directing pp28 to the assembly complex where new CMV virion progeny undergo secondary envelopment.

4.6. UL56

Currently, all of the licensed drugs used for the systemic treatment of acute CMV infection act through similar mechanisms as they target the viral DNA polymerase (UL54) [96]. With the emergence of ganciclovir-resistant strains of CMV, as well as cross-resistance to second-line agents (foscarnet and cidofovir), there is a need for new drugs [97].

A promising small molecule antiviral candidate, AIC246, is representative of the 3,4 dihydro-quinazoline nonnucleoside CMV inhibitors [98]. AIC246 acts through a unique mechanism distinct from that of the CMV DNA polymerase inhibitors. AIC246 blocks viral replication without inhibiting the synthesis of progeny CMV genomic DNA or viral proteins. Three pieces of evidence show AIC246 interferes with CMV DNA cleavage/packaging via a distinct molecular mechanism from other compounds that target the CMV viral terminase [99]. First, AIC246 does not affect CMV protein expression or CMV DNA replication, excluding the possibility of AIC246 acting through interfering with viral genome replication [99]. Second, genetic mapping of AIC246 resistance to the CMV open reading frame of UL56 shows that the viral terminase complex is involved in the action of AIC246 [99]. Third, a terminase cleavage assay showed potent inhibition of the formation of properly processed unit-length genomes [99]. Thus, AIC246 is a promising therapeutic candidate for the treatment of acute CMV infection through its unique mechanism of action involving the UL56 tegument protein involved in DNA packaging.

4.7. Antisense oligonucleotides

The expression of viral genes encoding proteins essential for the production of infectious virions can also be targeted. Fomivirsen, a 21-base phosphorothioate oligodeoxynucleotide complementary to the messenger RNA (mRNA) of the major immediate-early region proteins of CMV, can inhibit CMV gene expression through an antisense mechanism. Fomivirsen binds to the target mRNA transcripts of the immediate-early region 2 (IE2) that encodes several proteins responsible for the regulation of viral gene expression. This binding inhibits IE2 protein synthesis and the activation of immediate-early gene expression by pp71, which subsequently inhibits viral replication [100]. Fomivirsen is licensed to treat acute CMV infection and illustrates that CMV tegument proteins can targeted indirectly.

5. Conclusion

CMV infects most individuals by early adulthood and is associated with morbidity and mortality, especially in those with poor immune systems. Furthermore, CMV has been implicated in inflammatory and proliferative diseases, such as cardiovascular disease and cancer. Antiviral agents able to inhibit the CMV replication cycle and the production of new infectious virions exist, but suffer from high levels of toxicity and low levels of bioavailability. CMV resistant and cross-resistant strains develop because all drugs target the viral DNA polymerase UL54. There is also no vaccine available to prevent acute CMV infection. However, several components of the CMV virion are promising targets for novel antiviral therapeutics

http://dx.doi.org/10.5772/55156

that would inhibit the CMV lytic cycle and eradicate the virus from host cells. The most likely targets within the CMV virion are those proteins found within the tegument, which is a unique structure found in all members of the *Herpesviridae* family. Proteins that localize to the tegument play pivotal roles in all stages of the CMV life cycle. Novel antiviral therapeutics that target these proteins inhibit the CMV lytic cycle. Furthermore, the highly immunogenic nature of several tegument proteins makes them excellent candidates for subunit vaccines. In fact, several novel antiviral therapeutics and CMV vaccines based around the CMV tegument proteins are under development. Nonetheless, more research needs to be done to fully identify the function as well as the role in the lytic stage of the CMV life cycle.

Author details

John Paul III Tomtishen

Address all correspondence to: jpt015@bucknell.edu

Developmental Therapeutics Program, Fox Chase Cancer Center, Philadelphia, PA, USA

References

[1] arski, E. S., T. Shenk, and R. F. Pass. Cytomegaloviruses. In D. M. Knipe and P. M. Howley (ed.), Fields virology, 5th ed. Lippincott Williams & Wilkins, Philadelphia, PA; 2007. p2701-2772.

[2] Selinsky C, Luke C, Wloch M, Geall A, Hermanson G, et al. A DNA-based vaccine for the prevention of human cytomegalovirus-associated diseases. Human Vaccines 1; 2005. p16-23.

[3] Sinzger, C., A. Grefte, B. Plachter, A. S. H. Gouw, T. H. The, and G. Jahn. Fibroblasts, epithelial cells, endothelial cells, and smooth muscle cells are major targets of human cytomegalovirus infection in lung and gastrointestinal tissues. J. Gen. Virol. 76; 1995. p741-750.

[4] Steininger, C. Clinical relevance of cytomegalovirus infection in patients with disorders of the immune system. Clin. Microbiol. Infect. 13; 2007. p953-963.

[5] Rafailidis PI, Mourtzoukou EG, Varbobitis IC, et al. Severe cytomegalovirus infection in apparently immunocompetent patients: a systematic review. Virol J. 5; 2008; p47.

[6] Naucler C. Does cytomegalovirus play a causative role in the development of various inflammatory diseases and cancer? J. Intern. Med. 259; 2006; p219-246.

[7] Koch, S., R. Solana, O. Dela Rosa, and G. Pawelec. Human cytomegalovirus infection and T cell immunosenescence: a mini review. Mech. Ageing Dev. 127; 2006; p538-543.

[8] Grosse, S. D., D. S. Ross, and S. C. Dollard. Congenital cytomegalovirus (CMV) infection as a cause of permanent bilateral hearing loss: a quantitative assessment. J. Clin. Virol. 41; 2008; p57-62.

[9] Saffert, R. T., R. R. Penkert, and R. F. Kalejta. Cellular and viral control over the initial events of human cytomegalovirus experimental latency in CD34+ cells. J. Virol. 84; 2010; p5594-5604.

[10] Cinatl J, Jr, Cinatl J, Vogel JU, Rabenau H, Kornhuber B, Doerr HW. Modulatory effects of human cytomegalovirus infection on malignant properties of cancer cells. Intervirology. 39; 1996; p259-269.

[11] Cinatl J, Jr, Cinatl J, Vogel JU, Kotchetkov R, Driever PH, Kabickova H, Kornhuber B, Schwabe D, Doerr HW. Persistent human cytomegalovirus infection induces drug resistance and alteration of programmed cell death in human neuroblastoma cells. Cancer Res. 58; 1998; p367-372.

[12] Cinatl J, Jr, Vogel JU, Kotchetkov R, Doerr HW. Oncomodulatory signals by regulatory proteins encoded by human cytomegalovirus: a novel role for viral infection in tumor progression. FEMS Microbiol Rev. 28; 2004; p59-77.

[13] Melnick M, Sedghizadeh PP, Allen CM, Jaskoll T. Human cytomegalovirus and mucoepidermoid carcinoma of salivary glands: Cell-specific localization of active viral and oncogenic signaling proteins is confirmatory of a causal relationship. Experimental and molecular pathology. 92; 2011; p118-125.

[14] Matthews T, Boehme R. Antiviral activity and mechanism of action of ganciclovir . Rev Infect Dis. 10; Suppl 3; 1988; pS490-S494.

[15] C.S. Crumpacker. Mechanism of action of Foscarnet against viral polymerases. Am. J. Med., 92; 1992; p3S-7S.

[16] DeClercq, E. Therapeutic potential of Cidofovir (HPMPC, Vistide) for the treatment of DNA virus (i.e. herpes-, papova-, pox- and adenovirus) infections. Verhandelingen – Koninklijke Academie voor Geneeskunde Van Belgie. 58; 1996; p19-47.

[17] Biron, K. K. Antiviral drugs for cytomegalovirus disease. Antivir. Res. 71; 2006; p154-163.

[18] Kalejta, R.F. Tegument proteins of human cytomegalovirus. Microbiol. Mol. Biol. Rev. 72; 2008; p249-265.

[19] Shenk, Thomas, and Mark F. Stinski. Human Cytomegalovirus. 1st ed. Vol. 325. Berlin: Springer, 2008. Current Topics in Microbiology and Immunology.

[20] Chen, D. H., H. Jiang, M. Lee, F. Liu, and Z. H. Zhou. Three-dimensional visualization of tegument/capsid interactions in the intact human cytomegalovirus. Virology 260; 1999; p10-16.

[21] Varnum, S. M., D. N. Streblow, M. E. Monroe, P. Smith, K. J. Auberry, L. Pasa-Tolic, D. Wang, D. G. Camp, K. Rodland, S. Wiley, W. Britt, T. Shenk, R. D. Smith, and J.

Nelson. Identification of proteins in human cytomegalovirus (HCMV) particles: the HCMV proteome. J. Virol. 78; 2004; p10960-10966.

[22] Kalejta, R. F. Functions of human cytomegalovirus tegument proteins prior to immediate early gene expression. Curr. Top. Microbiol. Immunol. 325; 2008; p101-116.

[23] Adair, R., E. R. Douglas, J. B. Maclean, S. Y. Graham, J. D. Aitken, F. E. Jamieson, and D. J. Dargan. The products of human cytomegalovirus genes UL23, UL24, UL43 and US22 are tegument components. J. Gen. Virol. 83; 2002; p1315-1324.

[24] Stamminger, T., Gstaiger, M., Weinzierl, K., Lorz, K., Winkler, M. & Schaffner, W. Open reading frame UL26 of human cytomegalovirus encodes a novel tegument protein that contains a strong transcriptional activation domain. J Virol 76; 2002; p4836-4847.

[25] Zini, N., M. C. Battista, S. Santi, M. Riccio, G. Bergamini, M. P. Landini, and N. M. Maraldi. The novel structural protein of human cytomegalovirus, pUL25, is localized in the viral tegument. J. Virol. 73; 1999; p6073-6075.

[26] AuCoin, D. P., G. B. Smith, C. D. Meiering, and E. S. Mocarski. Betaherpesvirus conserved cytomegalovirus tegument protein ppUL32 (pp150) controls cytoplasmic events during virion maturation. J. Virol. 80; 2006; p8199-8210.

[27] Schierling, K., C. Buser, T. Mertens, and M. Winkler. Human cytomegalovirus tegument protein ppUL35 is important for viral replication and particle formation. J. Virol. 79; 2005; p3084-3096.

[28] McCormick et al. The human cytomegalovirus UL36 gene controls caspase-dependent and -independent cell death programs activated by infection of monocytes differentiating to macrophages J. Virol., 84; 2010; p5108-5123.

[29] Terhune, S., E. Torigoi, N. Moorman, M. Silva, Z. Qian, T. Shenk, and D. Yu. Human cytomegalovirus UL38 protein blocks apoptosis. J. Virol. 81; 2007; p3109-3123.

[30] Krosky, P. M., M. C. Baek, W. J. Jahng, I. Barrera, R. J. Harvey, K. K. Biron, D. M. Coen, and P. B. Sentha. The human cytomegalovirus UL44 protein is a substrate for the UL97 protein kinase. J. Virol. 77; 2003; p7720-7727.

[31] Isomura, H., M. F. Stinski, A. Kudoh, S. Nakayama, S. Iwahori, Y. Sato, and T. Tsurumi. The late promoter of the human cytomegalovirus viral DNA polymerase processivity factor has an impact on delayed early and late viral gene products but not on viral DNA synthesis. J. Virol. 81; 2007; p6197-6206.

[32] Patrone, M., E. Percivalle, M. Secchi, L. Fiorina, G. Pedrali-Noy, M. Zoppe, F. Baldanti, G. Hahn, U. H. Koszinowski, G. Milanesi, and A. Gallina. The human cytomegalovirus UL45 gene product is a late, virion-associated protein influencing virus growth at low multiplicities of infection. J. Gen. Virol. 84; 2003; p3359-3370.

[33] Bechtel, J. T., and T. Shenk. Human cytomegalovirus UL47 tegument protein functions after entry and before immediate-early gene expression. J. Virol. 76; 2002; p1043-1050.

[34] Kim, E.T., S.E. Oh, Y.O. Lee, W. Gibson, J.H. Ahn. Cleavage specificity of the UL48 deubiquitinating protease activity of human cytomegalovirus and the growth of an active-site mutant virus in cultured cells. J. Virol. 83; 2009; p12046-12056.

[35] Rupp, B., Z. Ruzsics, C. Buser, B. Adler, P. Walther, and U. H. Koszinowski. Random screening for dominant-negative mutants of the cytomegalovirus nuclear egress protein M50. J. Virol. 81; 2007; p55085517.

[36] Sam et al. Biochemical, biophysical, and mutational analyses of subunit interactions of the human cytomegalovirus nuclear egress complex J. Virol., 83; 2009, p2996-3006

[37] Kouzarides, T., A. T. Bankier, S. C. Satchwell, K. Weston, P. Tomlinson, and B. G. Barrell. Sequence and transcription analysis of the human cytomegalovirus DNA polymerase gene. J. Virol. 61; 1987; p125-133.

[38] Bogner E., Radsak K., Stinski M. F. The gene product of human cytomegalovirus open reading frame UL56 binds the pac motif and has specific nuclease activity. J. Virol. 72; 1998; p2259-2264.

[39] Kemble, G. W., A. L. McCormick, L. Pereira, and E. S. Mocarski. A cytomegalovirus protein with properties of herpes simplex virus ICP8: partial purification of the polypeptide and map position of the gene. J. Virol. 61; 1987; p3143-3151.

[40] Kronemann, D., S. R. Hagemeier, D. Cygnar, S. Phillips, and W. A. Bresnahan. Binding of the human cytomegalovirus (HCMV) tegument protein UL69 to UAP56/URH49 is not required for efficient replication of HCMV. J. Virol. 84; 2010; p9649-9654.

[41] Schauflinger M., et al. The tegument protein UL71 of human cytomegalovirus is involved in late envelopment and affects multivesicular bodies. J. Virol. 85; 2011; p3821-3832.

[42] Caposio, P., L. Riera, G. Hahn, S. Landolfo, and G. Gribaudo. Evidence that the human cytomegalovirus 46-kDa UL72 protein is not an active dUTPase but a late protein dispensable for replication in fibroblasts. Virology 325; 2004; p264-276.

[43] Siew, V. K., C. Y. Duh, and S. K. Wang.Human cytomegalovirus UL76 induces chromosome aberrations J. Biomed. Sci., 16; 2009; p107.

[44] Isomura H., Stinski M. F., Murata T., Nakayama S., Chiba S., Akatsuka Y., Kanda T., Tsurumi T. The human cytomegalovirus UL76 gene regulates the level of expression of the UL77 gene. PLoS ONE 5; 2010; e11901.doi:10.1371/journal.pone.0011901pmid: 20689582.

http://dx.doi.org/10.5772/55156

[45] Y., Qian Z., Fehr A. R., Xuan B., Yu D.. Human cytomegalovirus gene UL79 is required for the accumulation of late viral transcripts. J. Virol. 85; 2011; p4841-4852.

[46] Cantrell, S. R. & Bresnahan, W. A. Human cytomegalovirus (HCMV) UL82 gene product (pp71) relieves hDaxx-mediated repression of HCMV replication. J Virol 80; 2006; p6188-6191.

[47] Yao, Z. Q., G. Gallez-Hawkins, N. A. Lomeli, X. Li, K. M. Molinder, D. J. Diamond, and J. A. Zaia. Site-directed mutation in a conserved kinase domain of human cytomegalovirus-pp65 with preservation of cytotoxic T lymphocyte targeting. Vaccine 19; 2001; p1628-1635.

[48] Gao, Y., K. Colletti, and G. S. Pari. Identification of human cytomegalovirus UL84 virus- and cell-encoded binding partners by using proteomics analysis. J. Virol. 82; 2008; p96-104.

[49] Wing, B. A., E.-S. Huang. Analysis and mapping of a family of 3′-coterminal transcripts containing coding sequences of human cytomegalovirus open reading frames UL93 through UL99 J. Virol., 69; 1995; p1521-1531.

[50] Wing, B. A., G. C. Y. Lee, and E. S. Huang. The human cytomegalovirus UL94 open reading frame encodes a conserved herpesvirus capsid/tegument-associated virion protein that is expressed with true late kinetics. J. Virol. 70; 1996; p3339-3345.

[51] R, Mocarski ES. Cytomegalovirus pUL96 is critical for the stability of pp150-associated nucleocapsids. J. Virol. 85; 2011; p7129-7141.

[52] Silva, M. C., Q. C. Yu, L. Enquist, and T. Shenk. Human cytomegalovirus UL99-encoded pp28 is required for the cytoplasmic envelopment of tegument-associated capsids. J. Virol. 77; 2003; p10594-10605.

[53] Ahlqvist J., Mocarski E.. Cytomegalovirus UL103 controls virion and dense body egress. J. Virol. 85; 2011; p5125-5135.

[54] Wang SK, Hu CH, Lu MC, Duh CY, Liao PC, Tyan YC. Novel virus-associated proteins encoded by UL112-113 of human cytomegalovirus. J Gen Virol 90; 2009; p2840-2848.

[55] Hakki, M., E. E. Marshall, K. L. De Niro, and A. P. Geballe. Binding and nuclear relocalization of protein kinase R by human cytomegalovirus TRS1. J. Virol. 80; 2006; p11817-11826.

[56] Feng, X., J. Schroer, D. Yu, and T. Shenk. Human cytomegalovirus pUS24 is a virion protein that functions very early in the replication cycle. J. Virol. 80; 2006; p8371-8378.

[57] Feng, X. Characterization of human cytomegalovirus pUS24, pUS23 and their interaction. PhD thesis. Princeton University; 2007.

[58] Odeberg, J., B. Plachter, L. Branden, and C. Soderberg-Naucler. Human cytomegalovirus protein pp65 mediates accumulation of HLA-DR in lysosomes and destruction of the HLA-DR alpha-chain. Blood 101; 2003; p4870-4877.

[59] Gilbert, M. J., S. R. Riddell, B. Plachter, and P. D. Greenberg. Cytomegalovirus selectively blocks antigen processing and presentation of its immediate-early gene product. Nature 383; 1996; p720-722.

[60] Prichard, M. N., N. Gao, S. Jairath, G. Mulamba, P. Krosky, D. M. Coen, B. O. Parker, and G. S. Pari. A recombinant human cytomegalovirus with a large deletion in UL97 has a severe replication deficiency. J. Virol. 73; 1999; p5663-5670.

[61] Prichard, M. N., E. E. Sztul, S. L. Daily, A. L. Perry, S. L. Frederick, R. B. Gill, C. B. Hartline, D. N. Streblow, S. M. Varnum, R. D. Smith, and E. R. Kern. Human cytomegalovirus UL97 kinase activity is required for the hyperphosphorylation of retinoblastoma protein and inhibits the formation of nuclear aggresomes. J. Virol. 82; 2008; p5054-5067.

[62] Dunn, W., C. Chou, H. Li, R. Hai, D. Patterson, V. Stolc, H. Zhu, and F. Liu. Functional profiling of a human cytomegalovirus genome. Proc. Natl. Acad. Sci. USA 11; 2003; p14223-14228.

[63] Winkler, M. Interactions and functions of human cytomegalovirus tegument proteins Monogr. Virol. (Karger, Basel), 24; 2003; p113-121.

[64] Luxton, G. W. G., S. Haverlock, K. E. Coller, S. E. Antinone, A. Pincetic, and G. A. Smith. Targeting of herpesvirus capsid transport in axons is coupled to association with specific sets of tegument proteins. Proc. Natl. Acad. Sci. USA 102; 2005; p5832-5837.

[65] Sinzger, C., M. Kahl, K. Laib, K. Klingel, P. Rieger, B. Plachter, and G. Jahn. Tropism of human cytomegalovirus for endothelial cells is determined by a post-entry step dependent on efficient translocation to the nucleus. J. Gen. Virol. 81; 2000; p3021-3035.

[66] Sinclair J, Sissons P: Latency and reactivation of human cytomegalovirus. J Gen Virol. 87; 2006; p1763-1779.

[67] McLaughlin-Taylor, E., H. Pande, S. J. Forman, B. Tanamachi, C. R. Li, J. A. Zaia, P. D. Greenberg, and S. R. Riddell. Identification of the major late human cytomegalovirus matrix protein pp65 as a target antigen for CD8 virus-specific cytotoxic T lymphocytes. J. Med. Virol. 43; 1994; p103-110.

[68] Arcangeletti, M.-C., Rodighiero, I., Mirandola, P., De Conto, F., Covan, S., Germini, D., Razin, S., Dettori, G. and Chezzi, C. Cell-cycle-dependent localization of human cytomegalovirus UL83 phosphoprotein in the nucleolus and modulation of viral gene expression in human embryo fibroblasts in vitro. J. of Cell. Biochem., 112; 2011; p307-317.

[69] Sanchez, V., K. D. Greis, E. Sztul, and W. J. Britt. Accumulation of virion tegument and envelope proteins in a stable cytoplasmic compartment during human cytomegalovirus replication: characterization of a potential site of virus assembly. J. Virol. 74; 2000; p975-986.

[70] Sanchez, V., Mahr, J.A., Orazio, N.I., Spector, D.H., Nuclear export of the human cytomegalovirus tegument protein pp65 requires cyclin-dependent kinase activity and the Crm1 exporter. J. Virol. 81; 2007; p11730-11736.

[71] Tomtishen, J. P. III, Tegument Protein Subcellular Localization of Human Cytomegalovirus" Honor's thesis. Bucknell University; 2011.

[72] Tomtishen, J. P. III, Human cytomegalovirus tegument proteins (pp65, pp71, pp150, pp28). Virol. J. 9; 2012; doi:10.1186/1743-422X-9-22.

[73] Arnon TI, Markel G, Mandelboim O. Tumor and viral recognition by natural killer cells receptors. Semin. Cancer Biol. 16; 2006; p348-358.

[74] Schmolke, S., P. Drescher, G. Jahn, and B. Plachter. Nuclear targeting of the tegument protein pp65 (UL83) of human cytomegalovirus: an unusual bipartite nuclear localization signal functions with other portions of the protein to mediate its efficient nuclear transport. J. Virol. 69; 1995; p1071-1078.

[75] Gerber, M. Development of a therapeutic vaccine to prevent cytomegalovirus infection in transplant recipients. OMICS 2012: proceedings of the International Conference on Vaccines and Vaccination, OMICS 2012, 20-22 August 2012, Chicago, USA.

[76] Chee, M. S., G. L. Lawrence, and B. G. Barrell. Alpha-, beta- and gammaherpesviruses encode a putative phosphotransferase. J. Gen. Virol. 70; 1989; p1151-1160.

[77] Sullivan, V., C. L. Talarico, S. C. Stanat, M. Davis, D. M. Coen, and K. K. Biron. A protein kinase homologue controls phosphorylation of ganciclovir in human cytomegalovirus-infected cells. Nature 358; 1992; p162-164.

[78] Prichard, M. N. Function of human cytomegalovirus UL97 kinase in viral infection and its inhibition by maribavir. Rev. Med. Virol. 19; 2009; p215-229.

[79] Azzeh, M., A. Honigman, A. Taraboulos, A. Rouvinski, and D. G. Wolf. Structural changes in human cytomegalovirus cytoplasmic assembly sites in the absence of UL97 kinase activity. Virology 354; 2006; p69-79.

[80] Prichard, M. N., W. J. Britt, S. L. Daily, C. B. Hartline, and E. R. Kern. Human cytomegalovirus UL97 kinase is required for the normal intranuclear distribution of pp65 and virion morphogenesis. J. Virol. 79; 2005; p15494-15502.

[81] Kamil JP, Coen DM. Human cytomegalovirus protein kinase UL97 forms a complex with the tegument phosphoprotein pp65. J. Virol. 81; 2007; p10659-10668.

[82] Gilbert, M. J., S. R. Riddell, B. Plachter, and P. D. Greenberg. Cytomegalovirus selectively blocks antigen processing and presentation of its immediate-early gene product. Nature 383; 1996; p720-722.

[83] Spaete RR, Mocarski ES. Regulation of cytomegalovirus gene expression: α and β promoters are trans activated by viral functions in permissive human fibroblasts. J Virol. 56; 1985; p135-143.

[84] Salomoni P, Khelifi AF. Daxx: death or survival protein? Trends Cell Biol. 16; 2006; p97-104.

[85] Saffert RT, Kalejta RF. Inactivating a cellular intrinsic immune defense mediated by Daxx is the mechanism through which the human cytomegalovirus pp 71 protein stimulates viral immediate early gene expression. J Virol. 80; 2006; p3863-3871.

[86] Trgovcich J, Cebulla C, Zimmerman P, Sedmak DD. Human cytomegalovirus protein pp 71 disrupts major histocompatibility complex class I cell surface expression. J Virol. 80; 2006; p951-63.

[87] Hagemeier, S. C. Functional Analysis of the Human Cytomegalovirus Ul82 Gene Product PP71 Protein During Virus Replication. PhD thesis. University of Texas Southwestern Medical Center. 2007.

[88] Tandon, R., and E. S. Mocarski. Control of cytoplasmic maturation events by cytomegalovirus tegument protein pp150. J. Virol. 82; 2008; p9433-9444.

[89] Seo, J. Y., and W. J. Britt. Cytoplasmic envelopment of human cytomegalovirus requires a postlocalization function of a tegument protein pp28 within the assembly compartment. J. Virol. 81; 2007; p6536-6547.

[90] Johnson, R. A., Huong S. M., Huang E. S. Activation of the mitogen-activated protein kinase p38 by human cytomegalovirus infection through two distinct pathways: a novel mechanism for activation of p38. J. Virol. 74; 2000; p1158-1167.

[91] Yurochko, A. D., Hwang E., Rasmussen L., Keay S., Pereira L., Huang E. The human cytomegalovirus UL55 (gB) and UL75 (gH) glycoprotein ligands initiate the rapid activation of Sp1 and NF-κB during infection. J. Virol. 71; 1997; p5051-5059.

[92] Landini, M. P. & Mach, M. Searching for antibodies specific for human cytomegalovirus: is it diagnostically useful? When and how. Scandinavian Journal of Infectious Diseases Supplementum 99; 1995; p18-23.

[93] [93] Lazzarotto, T., Varani, S., Gabrielli, L., Pignatelli, S. & Landini, M. P. The tegument protein ppUL25 of human cytomegalovirus (CMV) is a major target antigen for the anti-CMV antibody response. J Gen Virol 82; 2001; p335-338.

[94] Molecular Characterization of the Guinea Pig Cytomegalovirus UL83 (pp65) Protein Homolog. Schleiss, Mark R.; McGregor, Alistair; Jensen, Nancy J.; Erdem, Guliz; Aktan, Laurie. Virus Genes vol. 19 issue 3 November 1999. p205-221.

[95] Phillips, S. L., Bresnahan W. A. The Human Cytomegalovirus (HCMV) Tegument Protein UL94 Is Essential for Secondary Envelopment of HCMV Virions. J. Virol. 86; 2012; p2523-2532.

[96] Lurain N. S., Chou S. Antiviral drug resistance of human cytomegalovirus. Clin. Microbiol. Rev. 23; 2010; p689-712.

[97] Schreiber A., et al. Antiviral treatment of cytomegalovirus infection and resistant strains. Expert. Opin. Pharmacother. 10; 2009; p191-209.

[98] Lischka P., et al. In vitro and in vivo activities of the novel anticytomegalovirus compound AIC246. Antimicrob. Agents Chemother. 54; 2010; p1290-1297.

[99] Goldner T, et al. The novel anticytomegalovirus compound AIC246 (letermovir) inhibits human cytomegalovirus replication through a specific antiviral mechanism that involves the viral terminase. J. Virol. 85; 2011; p10884-10893.

[100] Perry C.M.; Barman Balfour J.A. Fomivirsen. Drugs, Volume 57, Number 3, March 1999, p375-380.